I0474067

The Thought Leaders Project: E-Health, Telemedicine, Connected Health - The Next Wave of Medicine

www.thoughtleadersproject.org

Dedicated to Tiffany and Allison

Table of Contents

Preface

We live in a world full amazing people tackling incredible challenges in their daily jobs . . . and winning. What happens when leaders go above and beyond to share this knowledge with their peers? How will you take these ideas and build upon them to become the next thought leader?

Progress and positive change.

In this book you will gain valuable insights, tips, and actionable steps from your peers that you can apply today as each leader shares their unique perspective on the practice of modern medicine. It is our desire to share our experiences to help you transform modern health care.

Enjoy and remember... "Action is the true measure of intelligence" - Napoleon Hill.

Introduction

The phrase "may you live in interesting times' is reputed to be an ancient curse. Optimists would assert "benediction" is the correct interpretation. Curse or benediction aside, we live in interesting times indeed, especially in health care.

Technology advancements have transformed industry after industry, opening up new avenues of access and fundamentally reengineering and redefining the customer experience. Witness the banking, telecommunications and travel as representative industries remade through technology innovation. With the proliferation of online education, academia is experiencing a similar remaking. So too the advent of electronic trading of stocks, bonds and other financial instruments has provided at home investors with newfound easy access to the financial services industry. Technology advancements have even challenged traditional constructs of "work." Work was the place non-retired people went weekdays from 9-5. Today, it's what people do and increasingly is neither dependent on physical location nor constrained to set hours. Similarly, banking, booking travel, airport check-in, higher education, engaging in sophisticated financial transactions, etc. can now be experienced free of time and geographic constraints.

What of health care? Before our eyes, health care is being remade, rapidly. Why? How will health care evolve? When? What can we expect? What is the role of technology in the transformation of our health care system? Is the essence of health care and the doctor patient relationship so unique and fundamentally different from the industries discussed above that their evolutionary pathways are simply irrelevant to our American health care traditions and trajectory?

In this book, the authors attempt to address the questions above, suggest new ways in which you as a consumer might interact with your health care system and stimulate thinking, discussion and action.

With approximately 45 million Americans without health insurance, with US health expenditure rapidly approaching $3 trillion annually (translating into nearly $10,000 per person and 20 percent of our Gross Domestic Product), and with reports that in international comparisons US health care outcomes are not among the highest ranked, there is good reason to reexamine health care and challenge it - - through experimentation, free enterprise, and carrot and stick approaches - - to do better. In 2009 and 2010 landmark federal legislation, having a profound and long reaching effect on health care, was enacted. All of these factors are undeniable catalysts for meaningful change.

For generations, the provider has been the locus of care. Health care reform, changing and uncertain regulatory requirements, lower reimbursement rates and payment schemes that shift financial risk to providers have created business pressure and resulted in contractions in health care. The new normal is care redesign, health care business model experimentation, consolidations, mergers, acquisitions, divestitures, winners, losers and searching anew for cost containment and revenue opportunities. At the same time, a plethora of enabling technologies that has done so much for so many other industries have increasingly been applied to health care. Further, organizations not historically focused on health care have begun to look at this sector of the economy as a fertile market for their technology products and services. Before our eyes, health care is being deconstructed. It will be reconstructed and will be stronger, more efficient, of higher quality and deliver greater value. As the reconstruction occurs, just as with other industries, it will move inexorably to a distributed model with the person, not the provider, as the locus of care.

We are today at the earliest stages of this health care transition. Precisely how this transition will occur is anyone's guess, although it likely will occur in an evolutionary, not revolutionary, fashion. It is similarly anyone's guess as to the length of time it will take for this evolutionary transition to occur. Will it take five years? To be sure, five years is a long time and industries can rise and fall in a five year period. At the same time, five years translates to only five budget cycles and health care is the dominant sector of the economy. Great strides will be made over a five year period, but it is unlikely to be completed during this time. Likely, it is another continuous journey in the ongoing evolution of our health care system at-large.

Enjoy this book. Contribute to the discussion. Be an activist and stay involved in the evolution of your health care system. In short, stay connected.

Personally and on behalf of the publisher and the co-authors of this book, we wish you and all those you hold dear, robust good health and energy!

Joseph Ternullo, JD, MPH
jternullo@post.harvard.edu

Medicine Anywhere, Anytime: Disruption via Social Telemedicine?

Brad Tritle, CEO, eHealth Nexus; Director of Health Care Business Development, Informative Graphics; Chair, HIMSS Social Media Work Group

Telemedicine is an expanding practice in modern health care – one that could become so ubiquitous that it will lose the "tele" and simply become the average means of delivering medical services. Clayton Christensen, a Harvard Business professor, author and authority on disruptive innovation, terms telemedicine as part of the "second wave of business model disruption." Christensen states, "The second wave...will entail taking the solution to the patients, instead of taking the patients to the solution...connectivity in many instances will enable virtual decentralization – a movement commonly called telemedicine." Instrumental in this change is the use of social media, and the more private and secure enterprise social media – referred to as "the utilization of social media technologies in a private, behind-the-firewall, corporate or organizational setting." Current definitions of telemedicine easily allow the inclusion of social media as a delivery mechanism, and there are technologies and laws to alleviate potential privacy and security concerns with social media. By connecting patients and physicians remotely, social media applied to telemedicine has the potential to decentralize traditional means of delivering medical services and create an entirely new and innovative system.

Examples of Social Media and Telemedicine

Even though social media is a relatively new phenomenon, it is already being used by health care providers and consumers for the exchange of health information. For example, providers discuss cases through platforms like Sermo, QuantiaMD and Doximity; patients seek diagnoses, information and medical support through programs such as Patients Like Me and EmpowHER; and hospitals have begun using platforms like Yammer and Ozmosis. Though the intersection of social media and telemedicine is still in its early stages, there are several captivating examples that prove how successful such a combination could be in the future.

Type 1 Diabetes Application and Microblog

Dr. Joseph Cafazzo of the University of Toronto designed a mobile application and private microblog to help teenagers with Type 1 diabetes monitor and record their blood glucose readings. The application also allowed them to obtain rewards, such as games or iTunes music, for consistently taking their measurements. It was statistically shown that the program increased participants' compliance with such medically necessary tasks by 49.6 percent. This incredible example demonstrates how the utilization of social media can boost patient compliance and thus improve overall health.

SPINN Patient Engagement System

Another cutting-edge example is the SPINN Patient Engagement System's telemedicine delivery to Centerstone, the nation's largest non-profit provider of community-based behavioral health care. The SPINN system implements social media, secure messaging, video conferencing and interface capabilities so that Centerstone can engage substance abusers who are seeking help on the Web, but not receiving treatment. Linda Grove-Paul, Director of Addiction and Forensic Services at Centerstone, recounts the benefits of utilizing telemedicine for these services, "Social media offers the opportunity to lower the barriers to seeking help by allowing people to find assistance at their own pace using the tools that are a part of how they live so many other aspects of their lives. Social media, both as a point of entry and as a tool to support recovery, is rapidly becoming a key component of our coaching strategy."

Dossia Personal Health Management System (PHMS)

A third example is the creation of the Dossia Personal Health Management System (PHMS) for employees and families of participating employers. It offers personal health record capabilities that combine the concepts of contextual social media and gamification, as well as the option to choose a number of vendor applications from a "substitutable app marketplace" that have built interfaces to the PHMS. One of these vendor options is AmeriDoc, "a nationwide service provider of consumer-directed telemedicine which provides consumers with round-the-clock access to US-based licensed physicians via online video, telephone and secure e-mail using its proprietary telemedicine technology." Because of this program, employees and families participating in the Dossia platform have greater access to medical care.

Arizona Telemedicine Program (ATP)

The Arizona Telemedicine Program's (ATP) health care interprofessional team training at its T-Health Institute in Phoenix also includes a telehealth social networking platform. Students from different disciplines such as medicine, nursing and pharmacology are organized into groups using innovative software and a large video wall to test the methods and outcomes of interprofessional interaction. The social media platform enabled multiple participants from various locations to interact in ways not otherwise possible. Dr. Ronald Weinstein, founder of the Arizona Telemedicine Program and President Emeritus of the American Telemedicine Association, has been working closely with other leaders from the United States and Canada on a related initiative called "Collaborating Across Borders," which addresses the use of social networking to advance health care learning and practice. The program just held its third biennial conference on interprofessional collaboration, setting an example of its potential for future growth.

The Importance of Privacy and Security

Most of the telemedicine and social media examples provided thus far are delivering services within a closed system – a secure environment with privacy controls, such as a hospital's internal network or a secure (SSL-encrypted) Web-browsing session. Organizations hoping to engage individuals for the first time may begin doing so in an unsecure online environment, as long as no "Protected Health Information" is exchanged. Though some providers of telemedicine services (e.g. AmeriDoc) do not consider themselves a HIPAA-covered entity or business associate, many choose to be compliant with both the HIPAA privacy and security rules, in order to both protect the participants and garner trust. Organizations that are not HIPAA-covered entities are usually still covered under the Electronic Communications Privacy Act (ECPA) and a specific health information security breach rule, both of which are overseen by the Federal Trade Commission. Thus, there are ways to ensure social media is both private and secure when using it for telemedicine.

The Future of Social Media and Medical Care

With over one billion people using social media by the end of 2011, it would seem that the best way to engage consumers would be to further explore the use of this new technological phenomenon, specifically for the provision of medical care. Social media can beneficially contribute to telemedicine. Thus far, the uses of social media relative to telemedicine include enhancing existing consumer/patient engagement, acquiring new patients, improving medical education and practice and delivering medical services. But it is only the beginning. A variety of pilots, demonstrations and product launches will indubitably arise in the near future, bringing medical services to patients anytime, anywhere.

About the Author

Brad Tritle is currently Principal of Health-e Republic, CEO of eHealth Nexus, and Director of Health Care Business Development for Informative Graphics. His special interest is engagement of consumers through Health Information Technology (Health IT), for which he has contracted with the HHS Office of the National Coordinator, and other organizations. He was selected as Arizona Health-e Connection's first executive director in August of 2007, and led Arizona's Health IT activities for three years. Mr. Tritle is chair of the HIMSS Personal Health IT Social Media Work Group, Chair of the Health Record Banking Alliance Business Model Committee, a member of the Arizona Telemedicine Council, and active in both the Society for Participatory Medicine and the International Association of Privacy Professionals.

References

About AmeriDoc. AmeriDoc, LLC, http://www.ameridoc.com/about-us.html. Accessed February 17, 2012.

Cafazzo Joseph A., PhD PEng. *Innovation in the Medical Home: How Mobile and Social Technologies Can Accelerate Health Behavior Changes.* Patient Centered Primary Care Collaborative. http://www.pcpcc.net/webinar/innovation-medical-home-how-mobile-and-social-technologies-can-accelerate-health-behavior.

Cerner Makes Health Care Services Social with Jive. PRNewswire press release. http://www.prnewswire.com/news-releases/cerner-makes-health care-services-social-with-jive-125077304.html. Palo Alto, CA. Published July 6, 2011.

Christensen, Clayton M. *The Innovator's Prescription: A Disruptive Solution for Health Care.* New York: McGraw- Hill; 2009.

Collaborating Across Borders III. Arizona Board of Regents. http://www.cabarizona2011.org/. Last modified 2011.

Digman, Shane. *Can an App Save Billions in Health-Care Costs?* The Globe and Mail. http://www.theglobeandmail.com/report-on-business/rob-magazine/can-an-app-save-billions-in-health-care-costs/article2217094/. Published 2011.

Dossia Launches Next Generation Health Management System. Dossia press release. Cambridge, MA. Published July 20, 2011.

FTC Issues Final Breach Notification Rule for Electronic Health Information. Federal Trade Commission news release. Published August 17, 2009.

Grigsby, J. and Sanders, J. *Telemedicine: Where It Is and Where It's Going.* Annals of Internal Medicine. http://www.annals.org/content/129/2/123.full. 129, no. 2. Published 1998.

Hangouts FAQs for Administrators. Google. http://support.google.com/a/bin/answer.py?hl=en&answer=1261833 . Last modified 2012.

Healthcare 'Friending' Social Media: What Is It, How Is It Used, and What Should I Do? Healthcare Information and Management Systems Society (HIMSS), http://www.himss.org/content/files/HealthcareFriendingSocialMedia_AdvicetoConsumers_Final%281%29.pdf. Published 2012.

Hinchcliffe, Dion. *Social Business Holds Steady Gap Behind Consumer Social Media.* Enterprise Web 2.0. http://www.zdnet.com/blog/hinchcliffe/social-business-holds-steady-gap-behind-consumer-social-media/1695.

Levin, Gary. *Google Plus Telemedicine: Is the Patient Ready?* Healthworks Collective. http://healthworkscollective.com/gary-levin-md/28910/patient-ready-physician-20.

SGCL True 128-bit SSL Encryption. Verisign. http://www.verisign.com/ss/ssl-information-center/strongest-ssl-encryption/index.html. Last modified 2012.

Security Standards: Technical Safeguards. Center for Medicare & Medicaid Services. http://www.hhs.gov/ocr/privacy/hipaa/administrative/securityrule/techsafeguards.pdf. HIPAA Security Series 2, no. 4. Published 2007.

Serwin, Andrew B., Habte, M. Leann and Brown, Jerry D. *Privacy in an Interconnected World.* American Bar Association. http://www.americanbar.org/publications/gp_solo/2011/june/privacy_in_an_interconnectedworld.html.GP Solo, 28, no. 4 (2011).

Telemedicine 2.0: Connecting Medical Devices, Patients, and Providers to Improve Health. A TripleTree Industry Analysis, http://www.abl.org/Online/2007/050307/5-3%20TripleTree.pdf.

Telemedicine Defined. American Telemedicine Association. http://www.americantelemed.org/i4a/pages/index.cfm?pageid=3333 ., Accessed February 16, 2012.

Weinstein, Ronald S., et al. *Arizona Telemedicine Program Interprofessional Learning Center: Facility Design and Curriculum Development.* Journal of Interprofessional Care. 21 (S2), DOI: 10.1080/13561820701349321.

UA's Dr. Ronald S. Weinstein One of Three International Experts on Health-Care Education Reform to Co-Chair 'Collaborating Across Borders III. AHSC Office of Public Affairs press release. http://opa.ahsc.arizona.edu/newsroom/news/2010/ua%E2%80%99s-dr-ronald-s-weinstein-one-three-international-experts-health-care-education. Tucson, AZ. Published December 10, 2010.

Second-Opinion Telepathology Services for Cancer Patients

Ronald S. Weinstein, MD, FCAP, FATA, Anna R. Graham, MD, FCAP, and Gail R. Barker, PhD

Telepathology is the practice of pathology at a distance using digital pathology glass slide imaging and broadband telecommunication networks. Telepathology could potentially become a transformative technology which could provide a technical platform for the reinvention and globalization of second-opinion cancer diagnostic services. The goal would be to provide cancer patients worldwide, with immediate access to expert second opinions from highly-qualified subspecialty pathologists. Such services are currently available to a minority of cancer patients in the United States, and unavailable to cancer patients in many countries.

Gold Standard for Cancer Tissue Diagnosis

For nearly a century, pathology light microscopy diagnoses have been the gold standard for rendering tumor diagnosis. However, over the past 50 years there has been a growing concern over what is diplomatically called "inter-observer variability" in diagnoses rendered by different pathologists looking at the same histopathology slides. In lay terms, this means increased uneasiness about potential diagnostic errors. As better and more targeted therapies for specific kinds of cancers are being developed, an incorrect diagnosis might prove catastrophic for an incorrectly diagnosed cancer patient. Although the topic of pathology errors is handled gingerly by the medical profession, (i.e., "let's not cry fire in a crowded theater") before allowing initiation of therapy some of the best cancer centers in the United States now require new cancer patients submit to re-review of their original histopathology diagnoses by the cancer centers' own in-house staff pathologists. For example, Memorial Sloan-Kettering Cancer Center in New York City and University of Texas MD Anderson Cancer Center in Houston, Texas require that all new cancer patients send their pathology glass slides in to them for re-evaluation. In order to accomplish this type of comprehensive re-review of histopathology glass slides, these top tier cancer centers have hired many highly-qualified pathologists to perform in-house case reviews. Cancer doctors at marquee cancer centers know that laboratory diagnostic discrepancies (i.e., diagnostic errors) by outside pathologists can undermine their patients' therapies. As such, accurate pathology diagnosis is one of the cornerstones of the highest standards of patient care.

Very few cancer patients realize this is a problem area. In fact, relatively few physicians realize the significance of inter-observer error and the pitfalls of using histopathology as an absolute gold standard for medical imaging diagnostics. Generally, histopathology imaging is far more accurate than radiology imaging for rendering specific cancer diagnoses, but it does have its limitations as well. It is true for many types of cancer that almost any pathologist using a conventional light microscope costing a few thousand dollars will generally produce a result that is more accurate, sensitive and specific than diagnoses rendered by radiologists using million dollar imaging scanners. It is also true that in a large majority of cases, pathologists will agree with one another on a specific cancer diagnosis. Nevertheless, different diagnoses will be rendered by different pathologists in a small number of cases. A gold standard implies 100 percent performance and even diagnostic histopathology falls short of that mark.

As a practical matter, the large majority of cancer patients in the United States are not treated at one of the 66 National Cancer Institute (NCI) designated Cancer Centers in the United States. Because they're known for their scientific excellence, receiving the NCI-designation places a cancer center among the top 4 percent of the approximately 1500 cancer centers in the United States. The largest of the NCI-designated Cancer Centers have their own in-house pathology staffs, which does increase quality of care. These institutions have large cancer patient case loads and can sustain large in-house subspecialty organ-specific cancer (i.e., breast cancer, prostate cancer, etc.) pathology staffs.

In our experience, the larger NCI-designated Cancer Centers set the bar high for the best quality subspecialty cancer pathology diagnostic services. Achieving universal diagnostic services at that level of quality should be the goal for the entire health care system in the United States. However, variability in the depth and range of subspecialty pathology staffing in university medical center pathology departments can be problematic. In the United States, university hospital surgical pathology departments can vary in size by up to a factor of 10. Smaller university hospitals can be at a disadvantage with respect to the range of cancer diagnoses for which their pathology staff would have a high level of expertise. Non-university community cancer centers generally do not have subspecialty pathologists on their own staff, but outsource surgical pathology specimens for diagnoses. This can prove to be a disadvantage as it potentially contributes to the fragmentation of cancer patient care and might affect quality of services.

How can non-university community cancer center patients get comparable quality pathology second opinions in a timely manner? For many such cancer centers, unaffiliated with university networks, attention is given to making sure that cancer pathology diagnoses are being made by pathologists with high levels of experience and expertise in specific areas of cancer diagnoses. This concern for accuracy is reflected in the fact that individual expert pathologists, located in NCI-designated Cancer Centers or university medical centers, do render second opinions on thousands of cancer specimens from outside institutions each year. However, this is not true across the board. Many laboratories resist sending out problematic cases for second opinions because they would have to bear the costs. There are no regulations or guidelines that would ensure sending out cases for expert second opinions would meet a standard of care. From the patient's perspective, the processes are haphazard. Cancer patients rarely have any knowledge of their local pathology specimen referral patterns for purposes of second opinions or re-reviews of difficult cases. In fact, many cancer patients assume that their cancer doctor, typically an oncologist or oncologic surgeon, is rendering a diagnosis him or herself. That is a misguided and potentially risky leap of faith. The cancer doctor seeing the patient is merely passing along the information assembled by the pathologists who actually render the final diagnosis.

Fragmentation in today's health care system brings its own sets of errors, making it challenging for patients to reconstruct the pathway to their own final cancer diagnosis. In the United States, insurance companies have excessive control over the management of laboratory workflow, dehumanizing cancer care by creating barriers between cancer patients and the pathologist who actually renders the diagnosis.

As such, it's time to put a face on pathology.

Any assumption that all pathologists are the same is misguided. Commercial pathology laboratories often sell laboratory services as a commodity which doesn't factor in the individual variability of both pathologists and cancer patients. It should also be acknowledged that entry-level pathologists are often less skilled than experienced pathologists. Currently, the laboratory medicine industry is notably opaque. Patients know who their cancer doctor is but have little knowledge of the identities of the cancer doctors' supporting cast of subspecialty diagnosticians. Transparency is needed to enable patient participation in the selection of experts to render second opinions on the cancer tissue specimens. The lack health literacy on the part of many patients in the United States can also be problematic.

Telepathology is now envisioned as a potential solution to the growing need for patient access to higher-level and potentially more accurate diagnostic laboratory services. Two parts are needed -- a ubiquitous, standards-based telepathology service infrastructure and large-scale cancer pathology service networks. Several large companies, including General Electric and Roche, are developing and beginning to market industrial-grade internet-enabled digital pathology imaging systems for telepathology. At the same time, the creation of expert pathologist panels to deliver such services is being envisioned by thought leaders. Despite the great potential for growth within the laboratory industry, there are barriers to implementation of such services.

Histopathology Glass Slide Scanners Used for Second-Opinion Telepathology

Currently, the majority of pathologists in the United States have not embraced the concept of telepathology diagnostic networks. One reason for this absence of enthusiasm is the lack of familiarity with the latest advances in telepathology technologies. After all, the vast majority of United States practicing pathologists completed their training programs long before telepathology became available. However, pathologists would be well advised to examine growth curves for teleradiology beginning a decade ago or more recently, da Vinci robotic surgery for prostate surgery, to get some idea of the rapidity with which new medical technologies can diffuse out into the health care industry if they take hold.

Certain aspects of today's telepathology scientific literature reflect the recent growth of interest in the telepathology field (also called digital pathology, virtual microscopy and whole slide imaging). The scope of the scientific literature and the rapid growth of patented intellectual property related to telepathology and whole slide imaging suggests that there already may be a large reservoir of potential early adopters of telepathology technology into active pathology clinical practices. Clinical scientists who have participated in telepathology research practice pathology in hundreds of independent clinical laboratories located in dozens of countries. Thus, the stage could be set for telepathology, the service component of digital pathology, to expand into a global industry.

The scientific literature demonstrating the efficacy of telepathology is growing relatively rapidly. Nearly 1000 telepathology papers by over 2900 co-authors have been published in the medical literature. These papers show that the diagnostic accuracy of pathologists using this technology is acceptable for rendering expert second-opinion diagnoses. Telepathology also has been validated for use in surgical pathology quality assurance programs.

There are 78 issued US patents for telepathology. Large investments are being made in the development and marketing of whole slide image telepathology scanners. Well- established companies, including the General Electric Company, Zeiss, Olympus and Roche, have invested hundreds of millions of dollars in developing high-resolution glass slide scanners for telepathology and digital pathology analytical testing. These scanners are undergoing clinical trials, as a prelude to Federal Drug Administration approval of the scanners as medical devices. The slide scanner technology makes it possible to produce very high quality slide digital images of glass histopathology slides that can be stored on servers or in a computer cloud.

Of course, orchestrating paradigm shifts can be especially problematic and often have unpredictable outcomes. Telepathology involves a paradigm shift with respect to how pathologists practice their specialty. Instead of cancer pathologists physically peering through the eye-pieces of a conventional light microscope, computer-based digital pathology video imaging is used for examining glass histopathology slides. Digital image files are stored on a server and viewed by a cancer pathologist in virtually any location where there is secure internet access. Workflow software sends digital image cases to subspecialty pathologists with expertise in diagnosing specific types of cancers.

Telepathology is well suited to decentralization of the pathology workforce since pathologists are no longer tied to a light microscope and the need for hands-on access to glass histopathology slides. Ultimately, this could enable the formation of pathology "virtual" group practice networks across state lines and even international borders.

Telepathology as a Technology Enabler for Quality Second Opinions

As part of their quality improvement programs, many pathology departments have second viewings by a second pathologist of any newly diagnosed malignancy. In some practice settings, this process can be done more efficiently and at a reasonable cost by whole slide image telepathology. If this approach takes hold, it could usher in the development of numerous telepathology call centers, in some ways paralleling the current service offerings of many independent teleradiology call centers in the United States.

Doctor Reimbursement for Telemedicine and Telepathology Services

The stage is being set for reimbursement of telemedicine and telepathology services on a large scale. Some state legislatures have passed so-called "parity" legislation requiring equivalent reimbursement for telemedicine services and ordinary medical services. Although 13 states have adopted telemedicine coverage mandates, private payer reimbursement for telemedicine services elsewhere in the United States is variable and inconsistent. Unfortunately, some payers in other states have adopted the Medicare model for reimbursement. This inhibits adoption of telemedicine on a wide scale.

The Medicare program began reimbursing for telemedicine services in 1999, yet today Medicare only reimburses services on a small subset of Current Procedural Terminology codes (CPT codes) for patients located in specifically designated rural areas, performed by specific providers, using only real-time telemedicine modalities. Traditional CPT codes are used for billing and a telemedicine modifier (GT) is appended. Although a facility and transmission cost is reimbursed, the amount is so low (less than $30 per encounter) that it is not cost-effective for most hospitals to bill for the service.

The ability of the telemedicine community to increase services and relax current restrictions is handicapped by bureaucratic and unresponsive reimbursement processes. Within Medicare, getting approval for new billing codes has been a process that's moved at glacial pace. Less than a handful of new CPT codes are incrementally added each year.

The variability of state Medicaid telemedicine billing practices also inhibits a more widespread adoption of telemedicine. Although most states now reimburse for some telemedicine services, there are no standards or consistent practices. The result is a patchwork of Medicaid reimbursement models that are difficult to catalog.

One solution to the telemedicine services billing challenges might be to change how service delivery is viewed. For example, if telemedicine is just one component of a complete service encounter and not considered a separate process, the value of telemedicine could be significantly elevated through efficiencies, cost containment, and the decreased fragmentation of services.

Reimbursement for Telepathology Services

Telepathology service reimbursement is similar to teleradiology reimbursement, and some telecardiology reimbursement. These types of services enjoy a vastly different paradigm from that of other telemedicine services in the United States. The standard for telepathology billing mirrors that of conventional pathology billing practices. Pathology interpretative services, whether they are delivered by viewing images through a microscope or on a computer screen, are considered the same standard of practice.

Telepathology billing is handled in exactly the same manner as conventional pathology. The same CPT codes are used and there is no telemedicine modifier appended. Third party payers do not differentiate telepathology billing and reimbursement from conventional pathology billing and reimbursement. This is the universal standard for all payers, including Medicare, Medicaid and private insurance. The one disadvantage to billing telepathology using conventional billing methods, without a telemedicine billing code modifier, is that there is no opportunity to accurately report the volume of telepathology cases performed at the state or national level. One must rely on individual institutions to report telepathology usage.

Second-opinion telepathology (CPT codes 88321, 88323, 88325) is one of the most frequently practiced telepathology services in the United States. Frozen section consultation and diagnosis (CPT codes 88329, 88331, 88332) is another highly used telepathology service. Many other laboratory services are also successfully performed using telepathology.

Additional challenges to widespread adoption of telepathology services include equipment costs, appropriate specimen preparation at the referring site and integrating the telepathology service into the regular pathologist clinical service rotations.

Take Home Lessons
The road to establishing decentralized cancer second-opinion laboratory services has been long and arduous. However, the end

may be in sight. The laboratory industry is beginning to look at telepathology (i.e., the service component of remote "digital pathology") as a way to provide ready access to second-opinion call-center based pathologists. Although it has taken decades to develop and commercialize rapid through-put histopathology glass slide scanners, computer cloud services, and expert second-opinion networks, bundling of these components into viable services seems to be taking place at an accelerated rate. Instead of being frustrated over the current state of affairs in some areas of pathology diagnostics, technology and innovative ingenuity will ultimately succeed in developing new service models that will make readily-available, high-quality, second-opinion pathology services a reality. The vast majority of pathology diagnoses are already of high quality, adequate and appropriate, but there are clinical settings in which second opinions by experts turn out to be critically important. No patient should be blindsided by a less than optimally rendered laboratory microscopic histopathology diagnosis. All patients should be informed of the risks and rewards of their diagnostic procedures. Unfortunately, many patients in the United States would be unprepared to understand the meaning and implications of such risks and rewards.

In the United States, planners of next-generation health literacy education curriculum for K-12 students should be encouraged to develop learning modules on medical tests and their interpretations. Hopefully, the education establishment in the United States will begin to raise expectations for health literacy in the United States and encourage the teaching of medical sciences in both K-12 schools and undergraduate colleges. Access to internet health care education Web sites provides a starting point for patient education, but this does not offer a comprehensive solution. The answer instead, may lie in developing a multi-year medical sciences curriculum for K-12 students.

To reap the benefits of having patients interact directly with pathologists, radiologists, and other primary diagnosticians, the patients should have a basic understanding of diseases, therapies, and their management. Technically, pathologists could be reviewing histopathology slides with patients by telepathology if the patient had a fundamental knowledge of tissue histology and disease processes, topics readily taught to the general public. However, the current US education philosophy is that patients will learn about diseases on a "need-to-know" basis, typically after their disease is diagnosed. The United States education establishment undervalues medical science lifelong learning for patients. Unfortunately, this places limitations on consumers' ability to fully participate in their own medical care as full members of their own health care team.

About the Authors

Ronald S. Weinstein, M.D. is the Founding Director of the Arizona Telemedicine Program, headquartered at the University of Arizona College of Medicine in Tucson, Arizona. He is a Massachusetts General Hospital trained pathologist who for 32 years, chaired academic pathology departments in Illinois and Arizona,. He has over 500 professional publications on topics ranging from cancer biology to medical informatics. He has received many honors and awards for his contributions to organized medicine and for his innovations in the development of transformational health care delivery systems. He has received the Association for Pathology Informatics Lifetime Achievement Award. Dr. Weinstein is past-president of six professional organizations, including the United States and Canadian Academy of Pathology, the International Society for Urological Pathology, and the American Telemedicine Association. In the 1980s, Dr. Weinstein served as Director of the

National Cancer Institute-funded National Bladder Cancer Group's Central Pathology Laboratory and reviewed thousands of bladder cancer surgical pathology specimens from a dozen academic institutions for patients enrolled in cancer therapy clinical trials. This experience alerted Dr. Weinstein to the fact that inter-observer variability can be a significant source of errors in cancer patient management. Dr. Weinstein invented, patented, and commercialized robotic telepathology and is often referred to as the "father of telepathology." A popular teacher, Dr. Weinstein has received the University of Arizona's College of Medicine's Lifetime Teaching Award. He was recently honored as the University of Arizona "Technology Innovator of the Year." Dr. Weinstein serves on the Scientific Advisory Boards of DMetrix, Inc. and Apollo PACS.

Anna Graham, Ph.D. is Professor Emeritus of Pathology at the University of Arizona College of Medicine and Scholar-in-Residence in the Arizona Telemedicine Program. She has published widely on telepathology and telemedicine, including major papers on the validation of the diagnostic accuracy of telepathology. Dr. Graham has been a national leader in organized medicine and has received the University of Arizona College of Medicine's Lifetime Teaching Award.

Gail R. Barker, PhD works in the Finance Office for the Arizona Telemedicine Program and is a Senior Lecturer in the Mel and Enid Zuckerman College of Public Health. She worked on developing the Arizona Telemedicine Program's business model, has helped obtain third party reimbursement for telemedicine services in Arizona, and has performed a number of cost-effectiveness studies in the area of telemedicine. She is also interested in the use of technology as a high- impact educational tool in the K-12 curriculum.

Health Care in a Perfect Storm: A Time for Telemedicine and Health Information Technology

Dale Alverson, IT Medical Director at LCF Research, Immediate Past President, American Telemedicine Association at American Telemedicine Association

We face a time of remarkable challenges in health care that are striking almost simultaneously with amazing force, constituting a significant perfect storm. Upward spiraling costs and economic downturns demand that there be changes in and reform to our health care system. There is the need to consider new payment and reimbursement paradigms, such as pay-for-performance. There is the desire to put more emphasis on prevention, better health, and quality of life as opposed to reactive and procedure-oriented disease care. The general objective is to bring affordable, appropriate health care services to everyone, but at a time of increasing health care provider shortages. As the baby boomers come into the Medicare era, we also face an aging population with associated chronic disease.

Providers and health care organizations on a regional, statewide and national level are feeling concerted pressure to achieve meaningful use of electronic health records (EHR) along with health information exchange (HIE). EHRs can add value through integration of decision support systems that allow providers to manage the care of their patients with evidence-based, best practices while decreasing unnecessary variations in care.

Additionally, we are beginning to develop the concept of the patient-centered medical home (PCMH) to improve coordination and continuity of care that can include consumers' development of personal health records. At the same time, we are exploring models for accountable care organizations (ACOs) in order to improve outcomes, while reducing costs, repeat hospitalizations, emergency department visits, duplicate tests and medical errors.

Now more than ever, emerging health information technologies (HIT) and telemedicine will prove an important part of the solution in navigating this perfect storm by providing greater access to health care, improving health outcomes, reducing costs, and demonstrating a return on investment (ROI). This is the time for Telemedicine and HIT!

Telemedicine Blended with HIT

Telemedicine is the provision of health care services over distance which utilizes a spectrum of information and communication technologies (ICT) to connect health care providers. This technology can be used for increased communication between a specialist and a primary care provider or health care provider and a patient, independent of geographic and time barriers. These ICT tools can provide synchronous, real-time audio and visual interaction; video-conferencing; or asynchronous transmission of images for interpretation by a specialist, so called "store and forward;" or a combination of the two when evaluating and managing a patient.

Use of telemedicine can thus improve timely access to care when distance and ability to travel and related costs create barriers. Better access can improve health outcomes by providing the most appropriate care when and where it is needed, avoiding costly travel, preventing complications, and allowing patients to receive more services locally.

When a provider is evaluating a patient, there is the need for acquiring additional information, including health history, test results, and documentation of the encounter. Thus, blending health information exchange (HIE) with telemedicine encounters, becomes an important part of providing comprehensive care and management of patients through telemedicine, just as it is when providing care physically face-to-face. Together, HIE and telemedicine should be linked as part of an overall health care delivery system and enhance the ability to achieve meaningful use as defined by CMS.

Integrating Emerging Advances in ICT into Health Care

Wireless technologies, mobile devices (such as smart phones and tablets), remote monitoring, cloud computing, and other hosted solutions are providing new platforms that are improving access to health services and care coordination. These emerging ICT tools can combine EHR, HIE, images, video-conferencing, remote monitoring and trend analysis that will improve coordination and continuity of care, and integrate the patient more completely into the patient-centered medical home. Furthermore, as evidence-based best practices are incorporated, unnecessary variations in care can be avoided and the most appropriate care provided to the patient independent of location of the patient and providers. These applications of telemedicine should be customized to best meet the needs of the health care application, the providers and the patient.

There is mounting evidence and interest in the fact that telemedicine and HIT can enhance better care and health outcomes, while reducing costs and addressing social inequities of health care. In addition, accountable care organizations (ACOs), which are designed to improve the quality of care while reducing costs, can achieve their intended goals effectively by building telemedicine and HIT into their enterprise. Better care access, HIE, follow-up, and application of best practices can prevent medical errors, avoid unnecessary duplication of tests, and reduce hospitalizations and use of expensive emergent services.

International Development of Telemedicine and HIT

There is a global need and significant market potential for integration of telemedicine and HIT internationally. Using advances in ICT, telemedicine and e-health are providing a means to transform systems of care for people throughout the world by providing greater access to several important aspects of heath care, such as clinical service, consultation, sharing knowledge, education and training, public and community health, health systems development, epidemiology and research. Leap-frogging over prior barriers, rapid advances in ICT, computing, and wireless networks are offering greater continuity in access to these services in both developed and developing countries.

The use of telehealth must be put in the context of the how critical health needs are different depending on country, cultural perspective, current and future communication infrastructure, other supportive resources, and likelihood for sustainability. Furthermore, these telehealth efforts should be aimed at improving ongoing health services in each country by blending into that country's current and future health care strategies. In combination, these communication technologies and health-related applications constitute the concept of telehealth. As stated by the World Health Organization (WHO), to achieve the millennium development goals, telehealth is providing a broad spectrum of health services over distance and integrating telecommunications systems into the practice of protecting and promoting health.

Worldwide use of telehealth allows an enhanced means of sharing knowledge, expertise and evidence-based best practices, eliminating many of the usual barriers associated with distance and time. Global development and integration of communication systems and networks are creating opportunities for international collaboration using telehealth as a platform for exchange. Increased ease of global communication carries the potential for formation of a true "network of networks" and "virtual collaborator." A network of this magnitude represents far more than a communication infrastructure because it facilitates partnerships and collaboration between health care providers and educators, public health workers, investigators, and other international organizations and stakeholders.

As the world continues to "shrink," developing this international telehealth "network of networks" offers an opportunity for cooperation, collaboration and knowledge sharing which allows us to apply information technologies for peace and the betterment of mankind. The time is now for open and constructive dialogue designed to facilitate that coordination between key stakeholders and other international organizations. These types of international exchange experiences, enhanced with telehealth, offer significant opportunities for understanding the common denominators, as well as the unique differences, related to global health among countries and cultures around the world. These programs can promote international understanding and mutual respect in a manner that can improve the health of the entire global community. Such a significant change in the definition of a medical community requires thinking globally, but acting locally.

Adoption of Telemedicine and HIT as Part of Health Care Transformation

Diffusion and adoption of telemedicine and HIT will be based upon perceived value, ease of use, integration into workflow, and demonstration of return on investment. Organizational champions and opinion leaders will be important in convincing the decision makers of the value of incorporating these technologies into their enterprise. Therefore, it is critical that the ongoing research and data continue to demonstrate the value of telehealth in improving health, while reducing costs. With accumulating evidence, the day will come when telemedicine and HIT are fully integrated into a reformed health care delivery system and no longer considered as something unique, but as standard tools for enhancing health by providers, patients and consumers in general. If applied appropriately, telemedicine and HIT can assist in navigating this current perfect storm in health care and lead to new systems of care that will improve health and begin to control costs in a realistic, reasonable manner. The potential for telemedicine extends beyond the individual patient-physician relationship and concerns of a developed nation improving its health infrastructure to improve disparities in health care globally. Now, indeed, is the time for telemedicine and HIT!

About the Author

Dr. Alverson is Professor Emeritus and Regents' Professor at the University of New Mexico where he is the Medical Director of the Center for Telehealth and Cybermedicine Research involved in the planning, implementation, research and evaluation of Telemedicine systems for New Mexico. The UNM Center for Telehealth was given the American Telemedicine Association (ATA) President's Institutional Award for its efforts in advancing telehealth locally, nationally, and internationally. He is Chairman the Board of the New Mexico Telehealth Alliance and one of the founders of the Four Corners Telehealth Consortium addressing cross-border interstate issues. He is also IT Medical Director of LCF Research involved their efforts to establish the Health Information Exchange (HIE) in New Mexico, New Mexico Health Information Collaborative, addressing the advancement and meaningful use of HIE, adoption of electronic health records, and integration with telemedicine. He is a founder on the Board of the New Mexico Telehealth Alliance. Nationally, he is the Immediate Past President of ATA and has also been on the Boards of the Center for Telehealth and e-Health Law, and Advanced Initiatives in Medical Simulation. He is involved in several collaborative international Telehealth projects to advance Telehealth and Health IT globally.

References

Alverson, D.C. Telethinking .*Telemedicine Journal and e-Health*. 2007; 13(2):86-90.

Alverson, D. C., Edison, K., Flournoy, L., Korte, B., Magruder, C. & Miller, C. Telehealth Tools For Public Health, Emergency or Disaster Preparedness and Response: A Summary Report. *Telemedicine and e-Health*. 2010; 16:112-114.

Alverson, D. C., Holtz, B., D'Iorio, J., DeVany, M., Simmons, S. & Poropatich, R. One Size Doesn't Fit All: Bringing Telehealth Services to Special Populations. *Telemedicine and e-Health*. 2008; 14(9):957-963.

Alverson, D. C., Mars, M., Rheuban, K., Sable, C., Smith, A., Swinfen, P. & Swinfen, R. International Pediatric Telemedicine and e-health: Transforming Systems of Care for Children in the Global Community. *Pediatric Annals*. 2009; 38(10):579-585.

Alverson, D. C., Shannon, S., Sullivan, E., Prill, A., Effertz, G., Helitzer, D., Beffort, S. & Preston, A. Telehealth in the Trenches: Reporting Back from the Frontlines in Rural America. *Telemedicine Journal and e-Health*. 2004; 10(supp2): S-95-109.

Arora, S., Geppert, C. M. A., Kalishman, S., Dion, D., Pullara, F., Bjeletich, B., Simpson, G., Alverson, D. C., Moore, L. B., Kuhl, D. & Scaletti, J. V. Academic Health Center Management of Chronic Diseases Through Knowledge Networks: Project ECHO. *Academic Medicine*. 2007; 82:154-160.

Bashur, R. L., Shannon, G. W., & Sanders, J. H. (Eds.). *Telemedicine: Theory and Practice*. 1st edition. Springfield, IL: Charles C Thomas; 1997.

Bashur, R. L. & Shannon, G. W. (Eds). *History of Telemedicine: Evolution, Context, and Transformation*. New Rochelle, NY: Mary Ann Liebert; 2009.

Bashshur, R. L., Shannon, G. W., Krupinski, E. A., Grigsby, J., Kvedar, J. C., Ronald S., Tracy, J. National Telemedicine Initiatives: Essential to Health Care Reform. *Telemedicine and e-Health*. 2009; 15(6):1-11.

Darkins, A. W. & Cary, M. A. (Eds.). *Telemedicine and Telehealth: Principles, Policies, Performance, and Pitfalls*. New York, NY: Springer Publishing Company; 2000.

DeVany, M., Alverson, D., D'Iorio, J. & Simmons, S. Employing Telehealth to Enhance Overall Quality of Life and Health for Families. *Telemedicine and e-Health*. 2008; 14(9):1003-1007.

Frisse, M. E., Johnson, K. B., Nian, H., Davison, C. L., Gadd, C. S., Unertl, K. M., Turri, P. A. & Chen, Q. The Financial Impact of Health Information Exchange on Emergency Department Care. *British Medical Journal*. Retrieved from jamia.bmj.com. 2011.

Helitzer, D., Heath, D., Maltrud, K., Sullivan, E. & Alverson, D. Assessing or Predicting Adoption of Telehealth Using The Diffusion of Innovations Theory: A Practical Example From a Rural Program in New Mexico. *Telemedicine Journal and e-Health*. 2003; 9(2):179-187.

Jackson, G. L., Krein, S. L., Alverson, D. C., Darkins, A. W., Gunnar, W., Harada, N. D, Helfrich, C. D., Houston, T. K., Klobucar, T. F., Nazi, K. M., Poropatich, R. K., Ralston, J. D. & Bosworth, H. B. . Defining Core Issues in Utilizing Information Technology to Improve Access: Evaluation and Research Agenda. *Journal of General Internal Medicine*. 2011; 26 (Suppl 2):623–627.

Kaufman, K., Powell, W., Alfero, C., Pacheco, M., Silverblatt, H., Anastasoff, J,.Ronquillo, F., Lucero, K., Corriveau, E., Vanleit, B., Alverson, D. & Scott, A. Health Extension in New Mexico: An Academic Health Center and the Social Determinants of Disease. *Annals of Family Medicine*. 2010; 8:73-81.

Millennium Development Goals. United Nations. www.un.org/millenniumgoals. Published 2010.

Moya, M., Valdez, J., Yonas, H. & Alverson, D. C. The Impact of a Telehealth Web-Based Solution on Neurosurgery Triage and Consultation. *Telemedicine and e-Health*. 2010; 16:945-949.

Simmons, S., Alverson, D. C., Poropatich, R., D'Iorio, J., DeVany, M., & Doarn, C. R. Applying Telehealth in Natural and Anthropogenic Disasters. *Telemedicine and e-Health*. 2008; 14(9):968-971.

Tzeel, A., Lawnicki, V. & Pimble, K. R. The Business Case for Payer Support of a Community-Based Health Information Exchange: A Humana Pilot Evaluating its Effectiveness in Cost Control For Plan Members Seeking Emergency Department Care. *American Health Drug Benefits* 2011;4(4):207-216. Retrieved from www.AHDBonline.com.

Wang, C. J. & Huang, A. T. Integrating Technology Into Health Care: What Will It Take? *Journal of the American Medical Association*. 2012; 307(6):569-570.

Wootton, R., Patil, N. G., Scott, R. E. & Ho K., (Eds.). *Telehealth in the Developing World*. London: Royal Society of Medicine Press; Ottawa: International Development Research Center; 2009.

Health Care Roadway: Merge Right

Joseph L. Ternullo, JD, MPH, is associate director of Partners HealthCare's Center for Connected Health

Step-by-step, health care progress has extended lives, relieved human suffering and enabled astonishing feats not considered possible even a generation ago. With a professional culture steeped in discovery, NIH investing more than $30 billion per year in medical research, and vast commercial and philanthropic resources directed toward medical breakthrough, continued progress in health care is a certainty.

However, our focus here is on advances of a different nature -- those that endeavor to make health care more accessible and convenient. Can technology position each person, wherever he or she is, as the locus of care? Will this enable access to care whenever desired and wherever needed? In such a "distributed care" environment, how will the provider remain relevant? What effect on progress, cost and quality? Will new public policies need to be developed and existing policies reconsidered? In our time-constrained world, answers to these questions are equally as important as our tradition of biomedical research and advancement.

As we explore the answers to these questions, it's important at this juncture to define two common terms that for the purposes of this examination have very specific meanings. The term "provider" refers interchangeably to individuals and organizations that evaluate diagnose and treat patients. The term "person" refers to individuals who seek to maintain health and wellness, or otherwise seek evaluation, diagnosis and treatment for illness.

As has occurred in other industries, for the first time in the history of modern health care, one can imagine the construction of a 'health care '*roadway*' between the provider and the person, over which great volumes of health and wellness interactions will travel. Electronic in nature, the roadway will offer the person trust, convenience and value. These characteristics are essential to ensuring utility and adoption. For the provider, the roadway will streamline workflow, build capacity and enable new service offering capabilities. In this era of accountable care organizations, global payments and a rapidly evolving health sector, these features will establish the roadway as necessary to thrive professionally.

For health care at-large, the roadway will enable great leaps forward in efficiency and quality. New professional and paraprofessional fields will form. Novel research drawing upon the roadway's sprawling and unprecedented 360-degree informational repository will occur. Innovative health and wellness coverage offerings will shape ways in which providers and people engage. Novel cross-disciplinary collaborations between providers and organizations not traditionally thought of as health care-focused will occur.

Collectively, these changes will create new markets, build careers, inspire new fields of study, encourage new policy and culminate in relief of human suffering. With this ambitious and "good news" prognostication, the balance of this article provides a summary perspective on how, when and why this might occur.

Person

A fundamental goal for all of us is prolonged good health and robust energy. When illness comes, we seek a rapid return to health. When it interferes with our routines and disturbs our peace of mind, inevitably we turn to a care provider for support and relief – our doctor. The doctor-patient relationship, both professional and at the same time highly personal, is unique. Given its special status as legally protected and deeply rooted in trust and solidarity of purpose, even health care's most ardent critic and social gadfly would be hard pressed to refute assertions that the doctor-patient relationship is the one immutable cornerstone of our health care system, electronic or otherwise.

As one thinks about a roadway between the person and the provider, initially it is natural to envision a single go-to place in which all individuals interact with their providers. How efficient! Upon deeper reflection, however, a single, one-size-fits-all solution seems naïve and contrary to American-style health care and traditions. We prize choice, competition and free market entrepreneurship, and we are not constrained to one national provider or payer. It's hard to imagine how a single, go-to generic roadway gains traction and commercial viability. Who would invest the time, energy, thought and money to construct and maintain such a singular system? What would be the incentive to do so? Who would take responsibility when the system needed improvements or repairs? Who would vet content and take responsibility for errors? Why would providers sign on to an unbranded roadway, thereby providing an implied endorsement? What would stop the development of "private label" or hospital brand roadways?

A person's health status is deeply personal and no commodity. Divulging information about health and habits does not come easy. For these reasons, it is hard to imagine how a generic roadway could develop the depth of utility, personalization and customization needed to enable it to gain traction and achieve commercial acceptance as a viable pathway for interaction with one's provider. However, a provider-branded roadway rich with custom offerings tailored to individual health and wellness is vastly more appealing and consistent with our health care traditions, values and priorities. Such a roadway, offering the prospect of "wherever/whenever" access, builds on trust already present in our provider relationships and offers promise of new functionality and utility as our health care system evolves and modernizes.

Assuming trust is present, each of us will look next to the roadway's capacity for offering convenience, i.e., it must be simple to use and reliable. Indeed, there are models from other industries that can inform and guide roadway construction. Witness the convenience and simplicity offered by banks with online banking; travel businesses with online booking and airport check-in; financial service companies with online accounts; and telecommunication providers with bundled offerings. Convenience boils down to a simple computation of what health and wellness activities can be converted to the roadway and how intuitive the experience can be made for the users.

In addition to consideration of what current provider-patient interactions can be transferred to the roadway, due consideration will need to be given to design and usability. There are many qualified experts capable of convening usability studies, developing high-impact graphic user interfaces, and offering their considerable expertise and guidance. The existing industry skills and knowledge can be called upon to serve this inevitable provider-to-person roadway marketplace. Bottom line, innovations minimizing the use of time and energy and maximizing flexibility, freedom and independence will thrive. For this reason, a provider-to-person electronic roadway offering access to care when needed and where located will be of great interest to individuals indeed.

From the perspective of the person, the one remaining necessary component, of course, is value. What will go over the roadway, and how much will it cost? A plethora of activities will traverse the provider-to-person electronic roadway, some of which will be of no additional cost to the person, and some of which will have an additional cost attached. Activities traversing the roadway will evolve naturally over time. There are many likely candidates for roadway travel. These include remote registration and admitting; appointment scheduling for in-person and virtual visits; ad-hoc provider/patient remote check-ins; patient reading of medical records; automatic transmission of remote vital signs and other data into the medical record; automatic reporting of test results; automatic and customized alerts and reminders; health and wellness scenario modeling; push/pull access to clinical trial information; remote enrollment and participation in clinical trials and patient focus groups; participation in live and virtual patient support groups; involvement in clinical social media contests and challenges; opt-in reward and incentive offers; proactive monitoring of health and wellness data; delivery and viewing of patient education modules; discharge planning resources; pre-admitting checklists; satisfaction surveys; transition-in-care alerts; payer and pharmacy clinical and financial data; durable powers of attorney; informed consents, living wills and other advanced care directives; downloadable "apps," medical device plug-ins, etc.

While it will not replace real-time, in-person, face-to-face interaction with one's physician, the physician-person roadway will be a feature-rich, convenient, and adjunctive new avenue to access care, connect with one's provider and indulge in health and wellness. For each of us, the roadway promises to be our very own rich and robust personal health care "my-space" electronic connection to our provider. (Any similarity to the social media giant is purely coincidental.)

Over time the roadway will become a personal expert system about each of us and our health and wellness status. This function makes it valuable indeed and something that not many among us will want to dissipate or squander from disuse, misuse, underuse or peripatetic provider shopping.

Provider

The health care roadway will be a needed and welcomed resource to providers; especially as they care for larger patient populations and transition from today's fee-for-service payment model to emerging payment systems that essentially put providers on budgets and reward them for keeping patients healthy. Today, providers are in an "in-between" place as it relates to new payment models. Sooner rather than later, however, the transition will be completed and providers will have a newfound financial responsibility to ensure that individuals are well even when not in the provider's waiting room or admitted to the hospital and occupying one of its beds. That new financial responsibility surely will be daunting and pressure-filled, adding stress to an already stressful profession. It is also worth noting that the roadway will better enable providers to compete for and interact with the "Internet generation," a population that has come of age accustomed to technology, adept at remote interaction and demanding of 24 x 7 instant access. Simply put, the current demographic, financial and social phenomena change everything. They usher in a new era in health care; one requiring a provider pathway to the person wherever he or she is, whether at home, at work, at play or otherwise out and about living life.

The sheer intensity of a provider's day-to-day workplace pressures -- more patients (and demanding and highly informed ones at that), limited resources, constant time constraints, public reporting transparency requirements, and financial sticks -- makes tools that centralize workflow, provide structured pathways for self-care, and enable ready access to patients when needed not merely advisable but essential. Provider-to-person roadways offering remote triage and routing, patient education, shared decision support capabilities, and the ability to seamlessly add additional features in response to evolving needs and professional exigencies will become professional mainstays. In short, any tool that maximizes efficiency, automates process, enables people to achieve objectives remotely, meets legal/regulatory requirements, and is affordable and reliable will be essential to providers' daily clinical milieu.

A loose scattering of ad-hoc commercially available tools will be insufficient to achieve the utility and adoption contemplated above. Providers don't have the time to become experts on the plethora of commercial tools already available. Due diligence is required to ascertain reliability, fitness for clinical purposes, compliance with federal and state privacy and security rules, etc. To streamline workflow, ensure utility and facilitate adoption, centralization and standardization is required.

Other Stakeholders in the Health Care Ecosystem

While this article has focused on the health care roadway and the unique features and benefits to providers and those seeking care and health and wellness, the roadway will have a profound and meaningful impact on others involved in the health care ecosystem.

For example, it will create vast Greenfield areas that should be of keen interest to researchers and the pharmaceutical industry in particular. For the first time (from an ethnography perspective), we will have the technological capabilities to gain objective data and insight on one's health and wellness status where the person works, lives and plays. This 360-degree view should result in new and important clinical effectiveness and adherence optimization research inquiries.

At a micro level, it will create new areas of research for those committed to personalized medicine, as well as designer drug research and development. At a macro level, it will enable a deep and rich understanding of population health management possibilities as individual information is aggregated, trends are discerned, etc.

In at least two ways, the roadway will be a boon to insurers. First, it will enable the creation of accountable patients through access to continuous data gathered from all aspects of a person's daily life. The data can be mined and interventions and other incentives can be put in place to tilt patient behaviors in favored directions. Second, as individuals use the roadway in novel ways to indulge in health and wellness, data on what does and does not work will be accessible for investigation, early intervention and discontinuation or expansion of various payer feature offerings.

To put a fine point on it, for the vast majority of us, the grim reality today is that if heart disease doesn't get us, cancer will. We need new and innovative approaches to diagnose, treat, manage and eradicate the individual and societal debilitating menace that these diseases represent. The provider/person health care roadway provides an avenue for fresh thinking and new models of engagement that can be of particular benefit to pharmaceuticals, payers and others involved in the health care value chain.

Health Care at Large

Just as banks and depositors would not return to the time and geography dependent banking environment that pre-dated today's online banking world, daunting as the transition may seem, no health care stakeholder will want to forsake the benefits -- value, convenience, efficiency and quality -- of the progress that the provider-to-person roadway offers in favor of the status quo.

While the provider-person roadway shifts the locus of care from providers to individuals, it strengthens provider relevance, reinforces doctor-patient relationships and delivers value to the provider and the person alike. It creates efficiencies throughout the health care system and reserves the traditional office visit experience for those with a bona fide clinical need or personal preference for it. That's cost-effective capacity building!

It also creates a novel vista for continuous interaction, real time or otherwise thus enabling new clinical research of a dimension and in diverse settings not previously available. Further, the roadway creates opportunities for providers to engage in cross-disciplinary collaboration with telecommunications companies to build it, with consumer companies to design it, and with payers and pharmaceutical companies to study it.

The roadway gives new meaning to the concept of personalized medicine and enables discovery and medical breakthroughs tailored to individuals. Further, one can envision the creation of new classes of medical devices and point-of-care solutions developed for a world in which self care and remote care are prevalent. New professional and paraprofessional fields likely will emerge to monitor, evaluate, respond and otherwise assist the provider and the person with information traversing the roadway.

Of course, policy matters will have to be thoroughly studied and considered. Early participants will help to shape policy. Laggards will react to the policy shaped by early entrants. As policy is shaped, papers will be written and published, presentations will be made in public for a, and careers will be built. New coverage offerings, leveraging off efficiencies the roadway offers, will be developed, thereby enabling choice and liberating individuals to assemble a care portfolio meeting their individual needs. As more and more health and wellness activities travel over the roadway, provider/person relationships will deepen. Further, there will be a natural expansion of personal health and wellness information critically important to providers, individuals and to the advancement of health care. Paradoxically, this time of enormous upheaval will come to be viewed as one of the most exhilarating, innovative and productive eras in health care and will attract legions of workers interested in '*making a difference*.' The roadway represents an inevitable tool in today's technology armamentarium that promises to relieve human suffering, advance quality care and move healthcare forward.

Health Care in the Days Ahead

Technology has reshaped industry after industry and created new pathways to individuals, be they bank depositors, airline travel purchasers, or casual financial investors. That phenomenon has come to health care at last. Yet, to stand still is to fall behind. There are compelling forces in play today that point inevitably and inextricably to novel new avenues of access to care. As these avenues open up, they foreshadow great days ahead for our health care system and those who are part of it.

Ultimately, roadway standards will be needed.   Initially, they may be provider - - or regionally - -based. Ultimately, they will be global and constructed to enable local innovation to flourish. Eventually, with the advent of a flourishing technology-enabled healthcare system that places the each person as the locus of care, consternation about access to care, quality of care and cost of care will recede, and as a society we will go on to overcome other societal challenges of our time.

About the Author

Joe Ternullo is associate director of Partners HealthCare's Center for Connected Health and on the Northeastern University Health Informatics faculty. He's founder and organizing chair of the annual Connected Health Symposium, a preeminent international event for innovators operating at the crossroads of the Internet, mobile communications and health. Joe advises the US Commerce Department on international trade and the X PRIZE Foundation on its $10M Tricorder Competition for transforming health care. He sits on the review panel for the Office of the National Coordinator for Health IT's One in a Million Hearts Challenge and serves on the boards of Mass Technology Leadership Council, Massachusetts Health Quality Partners and Harvard Club of the North Shore. A co-founder of Continua Health Alliance, Joe holds degrees from Boston College, Bentley, Boston University and Harvard. He welcomes reaction to this article at jternullo@post.harvard.edu.

Is Telehealth a Reality or a Pipe Dream for the Private Practitioner?

Steven Hacker, Board Certified Dermatologist and Author of The Medical Entrepreneur Book

As technology has become mainstream and affordable over the last decade, "When will I get paid for using telemedicine in my practice?" has become a common question asked by physicians,. The answer may be "soon," or more cynically, may be "never." However, there are promising signs on the horizon.

The work of the American Telemedicine Association (ATA) continues to influence public policy and ultimately provide the data to validate insurance reimbursement for these very important health services.

In examining the reality of telehealth, it is important to cover the current state of outpatient telehealth services as it relates to the private practitioner. Additionally, it is critical to discuss the current technologies that make implementation affordable and easy, the allowable criteria for reimbursement, and the realistic issues that need to be overcome to provide, get reimbursed and implement telehealth services in a practice. Lastly, it is crucial to study the issues that policy makers need to address in order for telehealth to go mainstream.

Is Telehealth Technology Affordable and Practical to Implement in Private Practice?

For years, technology has been available to create a simple way to adopt, purchase and implement telehealth service in a practice. The best example of this is telemedicine technology which integrates videoconferencing into a medical practice. Videoconferencing technology has become mainstream, affordable and cloud-based.

There are now simple inexpensive systems that utilize a laptop, a high resolution video camera and the Internet.

There are also inexpensive systems that integrate wireless networking and robotics, thus enabling a private practitioner to be in two places at once, (such as in his home or office) and still visit a patient online in a remote rural setting, another physician's office, nursing home, or hospital. These affordable technologies which are easily and rapidly deployed, enable the physician to avoid the task of physically getting to the patient. They also facilitate increasing the amount of time that can be spent with a patient, and potentially enable providers to deliver certain services at reduced costs. The "robotic telepresence" that enables a "face-to-face" experience is available today. Systems may be employed using mobile robotic videoconferencing or even more simplified, fixed video systems or video cart systems. Integrated cloud- based commercial systems such as Citrix's GoToMeeting, Skype, or Face Time can all be deployed and configured in manners to respect privacy and confidentiality concerns with little to no upfront costs.

The benefits for the patients and the provider are numerous. In my own practice, I have used telemedicine to examine patients when I've been on vacation and needed to see a patient for emergencies, such as post-operative infections, post-operative complications and even shingles. Physicians can also make night and weekend visits from their home or office with the assistance of a nurse or an assistant who would be present with the patient. Physicians in private practice may see their patients when they are out of town, on vacation, or remotely from their practice for any reason. The challenges for providers to achieve rural outreach and the burden of travel time are almost completely removed. Rapid access to second opinions and in-home care and post-op monitoring become simplified and less expensive. All of this can be done in the name of better service, better care, and potentially a valuable revenue opportunity for private practitioners.

When Can I Get Paid for Telehealth Services in my Practice?

The Centers for Medicare and Medicaid Services (CMS) defines telehealth services to include those services that require a face-to-face meeting with a patient. The face-to-face aspect of this definition is relevant to the way that remote access medical services are coded and billed. For instance, remote non face-to-face services that use telecommunications, but do not require the patient to be present during their implementation, are covered and paid by insurance third party payors as if the service was provided on-site at the medical facility. These services-- such as a physician interpreting x-rays, electrocardiograms, or electroencephalograms -- are not considered telehealth or telemedicine by CMS and are billed, coded and paid as if the physician was on-site when he or she delivered said service.

On the other hand, reimbursement for telehealth services, as defined by CMS, is limited by the type of services provided, geographic location, type of institution delivering the services and the type of health provider delivering the service. It is important for the private practice to pay attention to the specifics of the CMS guidelines to ensure that it will qualify for reimbursement for telehealth services.

From Start To Finish Telehealth Service Must Meet Strictly Defined Standards

To be eligible for reimbursement for telemedicine services, the originating site must be approved by the CMS guidelines. An originating site is the location of an eligible Medicare beneficiary at the time the service is being furnished via telecommunications. This is very simple to understand, but burdensome to qualify for, and as of the writing of this article, an eligible originating site (i.e., private practice office for purposes of this discussion) must meet one of the following two criteria:

1. The practice must be located in a rural health professional shortage area (HPSA)

2. The practice must be located in a county outside of a metropolitan Statistical Area (MSA). (These areas may be found at http://www.census.gov/geo/wwwmaps/stcbsa_pg/stBased_2 00411_nov.htm)

The following originating sites, relevant to this article, authorized by law include office of practitioners, rural health clinics, skilled nursing facilities, hospitals, certain dialysis centers and community mental health centers.

The distant site practitioner, (i.e. the one providing diagnostic and therapeutic advice via a telehealth platform) must be one of the following: physician, nurse practitioners, physician assistants, nurse midwives, and clinical nurse specialists.

The last piece required to meet the criteria for payment for provision of telehealth services has to do with the technology. An interactive audio and video telecommunications system, (i.e. video conferencing) must be used that allows real-time communication between the physician at the distant site and the beneficiary at the originating site. *Store and Forward* telehealth (the taking of a digital picture and forwarding it to the practitioner not in real time) is permitted only in certain states (Alaska and Hawaii) and only for certain Federal telehealth demonstration programs.

The services that are eligible for reimbursement include consultation, office visits, individual psychotherapy and pharmacologic management delivered via a telecommunication system. These services and the corresponding Current Procedural Terminology (CPT) and Health Care Common Procedure Coding System (HCPCS) codes are listed below.

- Office or other outpatient visits (CPT codes 99201-99215)

- Consultations (CPT codes 99241-99255) Smoking and tobacco use cessation counseling visits (CPT codes 99406-99407 and HCPCS codes G0436- G0437) beginning January 1, 2012.

Other services that are less relevant to this article, but have codes for reimbursement include psychiatric diagnostic interview examinations, individual psychotherapy, pharmacologic management, end-stage renal disease-related services, individual medical nutrition therapy, subsequent hospital care services, subsequent nursing facility care services, diabetes self-management training (DSMT) services, follow-up in-patient telehealth consultation, and kidney disease education services.

Reimbursement to the provider of the medical services is the same as the current fee schedule allows for the service/CPT code submitted and provided.

Providers of the telehealth services must submit the appropriate CPT procedure code for covered professional telehealth service along with the "GT" modifier. The "GT" modifier is what indicates that the service was provided via an interactive audio and video telecommunications system. The key component that the provider must understand is that a submission with the GT modifier is mandatory, and its use indicates that the provider/physician is certifying that the beneficiary was present at an eligible originating site. If the beneficiary was not present at an eligible originating site, then the provider is not entitled to reimbursement for the telehealth service provided.

The strict guidelines surrounding the definition of an appropriate originating site keep telemedicine from becoming mainstream. Despite the efficiencies and patient care benefits of telemedicine, until legislation enables physicians to get reimbursed consistently in all patient care scenarios, telemedicine will remain a *nice to have* feature for most practicing physicians.

Once fairly compensated for their time and effort, physicians will be more incentivized to provide this service, and it will then become a necessity and mainstream. Once this issue changes, telehealth changes. It is complex because a variety of forces are pulling in different directions in an attempt to gain laxity on the originating site definition and criteria. Clearly, proponents of telehealth are seeking to expand the definition, but policy makers and budget hawks have different incentives.

Within the current CMS guidelines, a provider can generate additional income by claiming a reimbursement for a facility payment. This *telehealth facility fee* is billed by submitting HCPCS code "Q3014" and the place of service on carrier processed claims is code 11 (office). The office is the only payable setting for code Q3014. Again, once this code is submitted, the biller is certifying that that the originating site is located in either a rural HPSA, or a non-MSA county.

What is the Reality of Telemedicine Being Reimbursed in Private Practice?

There are currently twelve states that require all insurance plans offered within their state boundaries to pay for services provided by telehealth. It is the federal health benefit payers -- such as Medicare, Medicaid, TRICARE and Federal Employees Health Benefits Program(FEHBP) -- that are slow to cover services provided by a telemedicine program on a national scope.

The ATA has published "Six Fixes" on their Web site, detailing what improvements the current administration can make to advance health care delivery using telemedicine.

> 1. Mandate telehealth as a covered service under Federal Health Benefit Plans.

2. Increase federal coordination and influence on telemedicine.

3. Clarify that Medicare *Physician Services* include proven telehealth services.

4. Pilot telehealth service and payment models for Medicare and Medicaid patients.

5. Improve the process for CMS to add telehealth services under Medicare.

6. Support telehealth projects in the administrations FY 2012 budget proposals.

There are also numerous provisions in the new national health insurance reform legislation that may allow for advances in telemedicine. Though, as it relates to widespread use in private practice, these provisions fall short. The following is an abbreviated list of provisions related to Medicare.

1. Directs the new Center for Medicare and Medicaid Innovation (CMI) to explore how to "facilitate inpatient care....through the use of electronic monitoring by specialists based at integrated health systems"

2. Allows CMI as it develops new care models to explore how technology is utilized across various settings.

3. Requires new "accountable care organizations" to create ways to promote evidence-based medicine and patient engagement, report on quality and cost measures, and coordinate care through the use of technology, telehealth and remote monitoring.

4. Includes use of remote monitoring for eligible medical practices in the Independence at Home Demonstration Program.

5. Allows physicians to use telehealth to certify the need for home health service or durable medical equipment.

At the end of the day, we are still far too short on provisions that specifically address the ability of a private practitioner to employ telehealth services in practice and get reimbursed for it.

Legislation Needs to Expand the Definition of Originating Site.

It is that simple.

An expanded definition of the originating site will open the flood gates and change the way outpatient private practice medicine is performed. An expanded definition of the originating site means that physicians in private practice -- whether in qualifying rural areas or busy overpopulated cities -- will qualify for reimbursement. Reimbursement to all physicians for performing a telemedicine consultation, regardless of their originating site, will be the main driver of significant adoption of the technology. Technology is mandated currently on the data side through mandated implementation of electronic health records, but not yet permitted on the service side (through telehealth) in wide spread form. This is disingenuous, politically motivated, budget- restrained and hypocritical.

These two items -- the data side and the service side -- should be linked together, akin to a marriage partnership. It is inconsistent for the government, policy makers and politicians to argue for the adoption of electronic data and yet exclude the ability to provide services electronically through telehealth. The simplest solution for adoption of health records is to allow those physicians who adopt electronic health records eligibility for reimbursement of telehealth services.

In summary, the technology is available, the proven benefit of telehealth services for patients and providers is well documented (see http://www.ahrq.gov/clinic/epcsums/telemedsum.htm), but the policy makers are not yet ready to open the flood gates for implementation and reimbursement of telehealth services in private practice.

About the Author

Steven M. Hacker, MD, has extensive experience as a physician, entrepreneur and in the field of telemedicine. Accepted to medical school at the age of 19, he brings over twenty years of medical education and practical experience to all of his health-related businesses. In 199, he co-founded Skinstore.com (now owned by Walgreens). In 2004, Dr. Hacker founded PassportMD, a health, wellness and electronic health record company for consumers. PassportMD was sold to Mediconnect Global (now owned by Verisk Analytics, Inc.). Dr. Hacker has also served as a consultant for Fortune 500 companies, emerging technology companies, medical device and health care companies. He has published over twenty-five peer-reviewed scientific articles. Over the years, Dr. Hacker has been recognized by his peers with several awards and nominations including Best Physician Entrepreneur, as well as listing in Castle Connolly as one of the best physician's and dermatologists in the US and Florida. Most recently, Dr. Hacker authored a top-selling business book for physicians entitled, The Medical Entrepreneu; Pearls, Pitfalls, and Practical Business Advice for Doctors (Nano Press 2010). He is founder and course director of The Medical Entrepreneur Symposium (www.TheMedicalEntrepreneur.com).

References

Administrations FY2012 Legislative Proposals.
http://www.americantelemed.org/files/public/policy/SixFixes_Admini
strationsFY2012LegislativeProposals.pdf. Accessed 2012.

Mandating Telemedicine as a Covered Service Under Federal Health Plans. American Telemed Association.
http://www.americantelemed.org/files/public/policy/SixFixes_Manda
tingTelemedicineCoveredServiceUnderFederalHealthBenefitPlans.pdf.
Accessed 2012.

Medicare Coverage for Physician-Aided Technology Services.
American Telemed Association.
http://www.americantelemed.org/files/public/policy/SixFixes_Medic
areCoverageForTechnology-AidedPhysicianServices.pdf. Accessed
2012.

Medicare Payment of Telemedicine and Telehealth Services. American Telemed Association.
http://www.americantelemed.org/files/public/policy/MedicareTelem
edicine2012.pdf. Accessed 2012.

National Health Reform Timeline and Telemedicine. American Telemed Association.
http://media.americantelemed.org/policy/HealthReformTimelineAnd
Telemedicine.pdf. Accessed 2012.

Public Policy. American Telemed Association.
http://www.americantelemed.org/i4a/pages/index.cfm?pageid=3337
.

Six Fixes the Administration Can Make to Improve Health Care Delivery Using Telemedicine. American Telemed Association. http://www.americantelemed.org/files/public/policy/SIX%20FIXES.pd f. Accessed 2012.

Telemedicine in US National Health Reform. American Telemed Association.http://www.americantelemed.org/files/public/policy/Tel emedicine%20in%20National%20Health%20Reform.pdf. Accessed 2012.

Telemedicine: A Virtual Transformation of Health Care

Ron Pion, Clinical Professor at the UCLA School of Medicine and Sophie Shulman, graduate from the University of California, Davis

The term "telemedicine" is unfamiliar to most, but its concept is not as revolutionary as one might think. Technology has touched nearly every area of modern life. We have seen the Internet take society by storm, vastly transforming social interaction, shopping, education and music. In most cases, technology has made services faster, cheaper and better. People can chat via online forums in real time, an item can be purchased from one's couch in a matter of seconds and people can video Skype across the world.

But the industry that has arguably been the least affected is health care. Despite our advancements, a patient still cannot pick up the phone and speak with a doctor about a medical issue. It takes scheduled appointments, allotted time and high fees to consult a doctor, even if the issue is relatively minor. Furthermore, doctors' emphasized responsibility is treating the sick, rather than keeping people well.

Modern technology has given us an incredible opportunity to transform the health care system and the health of individuals for the better. Simply put, telemedicine is the use of technology to deliver medical services from a distance, but it is so much more. It is a way to collect data, distribute information and connect doctors and patients. When doctors can reach patients faster, their services are more efficient. When patients have access to medical advice and knowledge, they are better able to manage their own health. Telemedicine provides us with a great web of connection and resources we can use to learn from the past and each other in order to create a healthier present and future.

Return to a Simpler Time

Until the late 1940s, a significant number of doctors made house calls. Today the idea of a house call might seem like ancient practice, but when stripped down to its basic concept, it makes quite a lot of sense. With a house call, the ill person remains in bed, where undoubtedly he or she should stay to get well, while the more able doctor travels to deliver his or her services. In the current system, a doctor's visit requires an appointment, forms, insurance and a trip to the doctor's office. While one might argue that these may be necessary for our health care system to function in an organized and distinct way, the underlying purpose – to cure the ill – is not well served by the system.

Telemedicine can produce the same benefits of house calls but at a more advanced level. Technology, such as Skype and telephones, allows us to cross great distances in a matter of seconds, eliminating the need for travel by patients or doctors. Doctors could consult with a patient via Skype or phone without removing the patient from his or her place of rest, just like a house call. Furthermore, doctors can reach patients in rural areas that might not have access to medical services. By bridging geographic distances, telemedicine saves time, benefitting both doctors and patients.

Enhancing Quality of Care

In addition to crossing geographic distances and expanding access to medical care, telemedicine can also enhance the quality of care by delivering important medical information and resources to patients. The resulting ease and clarity of communication allows them to have an increased ability to monitor their own health.

For example, health education via a technological medium can boost patient involvement. One such service, Health Nuts Media, educates youth and adults about health and nutrition through animation, games and applications, encouraging increased involvement in health choices and outcomes. Often, medical terminology and processes can be confusing and intimidating, but by utilizing a fun, familiar medium to communicate these concepts, patients can better understand how to manage their own health.

Telemedicine can also provide patients with quick and easy access to their own health records. Surprisingly, most patients do not have ready access to their own health records. If they did, patients would have the opportunity to control their medical care more easily. The tools for healthy living would fall into patients' hands and doctors could focus less on treating the sick and more on keeping people alive and well. Perhaps it would force people to take health out of the realm of medicine, and redirect it to their daily lives at home with proper nutrition and healthy habits.

Furthermore, because technology makes communicating across distances easy, patients who are experiencing similar medical issues can connect and learn from one another. For example, a patient just diagnosed with diabetes can call or Skype with another patient who has been living with diabetes for years. The new patient can learn how to live successfully with diabetes from someone who has experienced it firsthand. Thus, a patient can learn and improve on his or her own without involvement from a doctor. If patients had more knowledge and greater ability to manage their own health, they would be healthier and save money, and doctors would have more time and resources to address more serious medical needs.

A Promising Future
Telemedicine is gaining steam in the health care industry. Two examples, Specialists On Call™ and IDEAL LIFE®, have recently made waves and have set a precedent for what can be achieved through the blending of technology and medicine.

Specialists On Call was created in response to the national specialty physician shortage, providing inexpensive and accessible emergency telemedicine consultations in teleneurology and telepsychiatry. Reports indicate over 33 percent of hospitals in the United States pay a costly fee for on-call specialists and that by the year 2020, the country will face a shortfall of 27,000 medical specialists. By providing services from a distance, Specialists On Call can reach thousands of patients in the Emergency Room of a hospital.

The process is simple and effective. An ER physician calls the operations center and an on-call neurologist is guaranteed to return the call within 15 minutes. The patient's medical data are delivered to the neurologist and his or her case is discussed with an attending physician.Then, a detailed consultation report is sent to the ER physician within 30 minutes.

Specialists are board certified physicians with the most current medical knowledge in their fields. The technology they use is secure and reliable videoconferencing equipment, along with HIPAA- and HITECH-compliant data and image management platforms. Data, such as patient records, is collected and stored in a secure database that is easy and quick to access. The primary focus of Specialists On Call is excellent care for patients, and they guarantee consultation within 15 minutes of a request for neurology and 60 minutes for psychiatry.

Post-consultation studies reveal a higher patient satisfaction than those who received hospital consultations. Hospitals also benefit because it solves the shortage of on-call specialists and provides more medical support at a lower cost. Thus far, Specialists On Call has delivered more than 25,000 emergency neurology consultations in approximately 200 hospitals nationwide. It is the first service of its kind to earn Joint Commission accreditation.

IDEAL LIFE was designed for patients who are suffering from chronic conditions such as congestive heart failure, diabetes and obesity, IDEAL LIFE supplies technological products that improve health. For example, the Gluco-Manager automatically captures, stores and sends glucose levels to the patient's health care team while the SpO2-Manager measures oxygen saturation and heart rate. All products are compact and easy to use, offering patients the convenient ability to regulate their health at the touch of a button. These devices examplify the use of technology to place the patient at the center of control, by providing monitoring on a daily basis, if deemed necessary.

Potential Challenges for Telemedicine

Change is difficult. Unfamiliar concepts, especially if applied to a complex system dominated by long-held practices, might not initially be well received. But our health care system has not been without its revolutionary transformations that have been successfully integrated in the past. The implementation of Medicare in 1965, for example, guaranteed health care to Americans over the age of 65 and those with permanent disabilities. Before Medicare, health insurance was either unavailable or unaffordable for most of the older adult population. Now, regardless of medical history or income, these groups have access to medical services. They do not have to hesitate before going to the doctor's office or consulting their physician. Medicare has made it easier for the elderly and disabled to receive medical care. Additionally, not too long ago, the Internet, Twitter and Facebook were new and unfamiliar, but within a short period of time they have become commonplace. Even older generations have embraced such modern systems and devices.

Can we embrace technological advancements that will benefit the medical industry in a manner similar to other industries? Can we guarantee access to the entire population, even those in hard-to-reach rural areas? Modern technology would seem to answer these questions "yes." However, it requires an open mind and determination to learn a new and unfamiliar system. If an 82-year-old grandmother who was raised without a television or telephone can communicate via e-mail, why can't doctors learn to communicate with patients through a technological medium?

Advancing to a Better Future

The ability to adapt to change is innate, but the capacity for high-level learning is a human power. In order to advance to a better future in health care, we need to examine past successes and combine those lessons with current advancements. If we take the simple concepts of house calls and the telephone, integrate them with modern technology and implement them into our health care system, we would see incredible results. Telemedicine bridges gaps – doctors can consult with other doctors across the country, and patients in rural areas can receive care and information. Suddenly, the medical world is not so large and unattainable, but rich with immediate access to knowledge and resources. Technology provides us with a tremendous advantage – one that is already recognized in other industries and sure to develop further into the field of medicine in the near future.

About the Authors

Dr. Pion is a clinical professor at the UCLA School of Medicine and a Fellow of the American College of Obstetricians and Gynecologists. He began pursuing health care telecommunications full-time in 1979. He is currently the Strategic Advisor for Specialists on Call, Health Nuts Media, and other potentially collaborative organizations. He was the medical correspondent for KNBC's Alice and Well news feature in Los Angeles. He served on the board of the American Academy of Home Care Physicians, the Abbey Healthcare Group and co-authored a book about caring for patients at home.

Sophie Shulman is a graduate from the University of California, Davis, where she earned a BA in Sociology and Communication. She currently resides in San Francisco and works as an integral part of the sales and editorial team at Marin Magazine and as a freelance writer.

Medical Innovation is Health Care Reform...or It Should Be

Joel E. Barthelemy, Managing Director, GlobalMed

It is widely accepted by people of various political persuasions that the current health care system in the United States is *broken*. Indeed, there are many challenges inherent in the way that health care is provided in our country, including an outdated, state-by-state licensure system, a fee-for-service business/reimbursement payment model, and a shortage of primary and specialty care practicing physicians in rural areas.

The Patient Protection and Affordable Care Act (PPACA), passed by mostly party-line votes in the United States House of Representative and Senate in 2009-2010, was signed into law by President Barack Obama on March 23, 2010. It is referred to by critics derisively as "Obamacare" and defended by proponents for various provisions it contains. One such provision is the one that stipulates that as of January 1, 2014, insurance companies cannot refuse to insure a person who has a pre-existing condition and has been uninsured for at least six months.

By the time this article is published, the Supreme Court may have ruled on the constitutionality of certain parts of the PPACA. But whether or not you support the PPACA, there are some areas upon which most can agree in the ongoing health care debate. Any kind of serious reform will have to incorporate technological innovations if we hope to achieve success in the goals of providing access to most, if not all, controlling costs, and improving patient satisfaction. Because many of the fixes needed could be accomplished easily and even inexpensively, it is surprising that there hasn't been more outrage expressed on the topic. Some of the answers are clear and ready to be implemented whenever we, as a nation, are ready to seriously tackle the problem. Those answers revolve around innovation and proven solutions. I am firmly convinced the future of health care in our nation lies in reform centered around advances in technology – not on more governmental fees on devices, taxation, regulation or rationing of health care. Allowing our most creative minds to run free to imagine, develop and implement new technologies will benefit us all.

The "Cloud" and Medicine

The "cloud" has become a ubiquitous term which refers to a set of technologies that enable the delivery of computing services over the Internet in real-time, allowing end-users instant access to data and applications from any device with internet access. Several real-time health care system delivery companies already deploy data and images to and from the "cloud," providing access anywhere for patients and doctors. This capability has resulted in saved lives and reduced costs. These software and service solutions, including some hardware devices, enable leading health care professionals to be more effective, more productive, and more efficient. For example, many of us have elderly relatives living in other states, oftentimes even across the country. What would you do if you were in Minneapolis and received a phone call from a doctor in Phoenix informing you that your mother was in the hospital? If the doctor asked you for a current list of your mother's medications and allergies, would you be able to provide an answer quickly? If that vital information could be stored in the "cloud" and easily accessed by the doctor, would you consider that to be a good thing? I think most people would answer "yes" to that question.

Electronic Medical Records (EMR), which allow physicians and other medical professionals to safely store your Personal Health Information (PHI) in a digital format, make critical information easily accessible when it is needed. EMR are a vital component in ensuring medicine keeps pace with technological advancements. Most

Americans realize the importance of widespread use of EMR technology. According to a 2010 Harris Poll, four in five Americans believe that any doctor treating them should have instant access to their medical record online

Defining Telemedicine -- Medicine at a Distance

Telemedicine, as defined by the American Telemedicine Association (ATA), is the use of medical information exchanged from one site to another via electronic communications to improve patients' health status. Closely associated with telemedicine is the term "telehealth," which is often used to encompass a broader definition of remote health care that does not always involve clinical services. Videoconferencing, transmission of still images, e-health including patient portals, remote monitoring of vital signs, continuing medical education and nursing call centers are all considered part of telemedicine and telehealth.

As our nation has been embroiled in a partisan debate over what health care will be like in the future, all sides agree that telemedicine should be a key component in achieving a health care system which is more responsive to patient needs and furthers the mission of physicians to provide the best health care possible at the lowest possible price. I am not alone in the belief that it is the "next frontier" in health care. One recent study determined that the telehealth market, which includes telemedicine and home health passive monitoring, is on track to become more than a six-billion-dollar industry by the turn of the next decade.

Listening and responding to the needs of their customers, forward-thinking companies are designing, integrating and scaling interoperable medical devices and technology into telemedicine solutions. If you lived in rural American town, such as Sweetwater Tennessee, and you suffered what an ER doctor believed to be a stroke, your rural hospital more than likely would not have a neurologist available to diagnose your condition within the critical three-hour window needed to provide aggressive stroke treatment. You would most likely be transported to Knoxville for the proper diagnosis and treatment, hopefully before the time that your outcome would be irreversible. However, with simple, secure telemedicine technology in that rural hospital emergency department and an agreement with a provider network at which a qualified neurologist resides, immediate access to the necessary care could be provided prior to transport, saving precious time, resources and potentially your life. Of course, there are regulatory barriers to be considered, yet despite their being erected to protect the public, people are beginning to understand these restrictions are isolating them from health care professionals. Consumers are starting to ask why more isn't being done with smart phones, tablets and computers.

Battlefield and Other Military Applications for Telemedicine

What is the future of telemedicine as far as the military is concerned? Recent events at Fort Hood and in Afghanistan would suggest military doctors must gear qualified care towards 24/7 accessibility for our troops, no matter where that doctor is at any particular moment. "Meaningful use" will combine Electronic Health Records (EHR), and its related technology to create a viable structure with the goal of providing cutting-edge health care to our men and women in uniform, here at home and on the field of battle.

We live in truly exhilarating times when it comes to the field of medicine empowered through innovative technologies. There are groundbreaking advances being made on a consistent basis which have exciting applications for the military. The day will come when medics routinely use a camera-type phone app to diagnose a wounded soldier on the front line, electronically transmitting information to other medical personnel hundreds or even thousands of miles away. With new technology, it is possible even now to do that on a helicopter transporting a wounded soldier to safety. It is truly amazing and useful technology for the military, which hopefully will be available soon for civilian medical air transports.

The Department of Veterans Affairs is one of the largest single payer/provider health care systems in the world. In recent years, the VA has invested heavily in a telemedicine program to serve our nations valued veterans and they are seeing a return on that investment. According to an article in *InformationWeek,* based on initial data in January of 2012 from only one of the VA's 23 Veterans Integrated Service Networks (VISNs), the telemedicine rollout trimmed approximately $742,000 from its budget during the same period by facilitating 23,580 remote consultations. Many health care organizations, including the VA, are transforming before our very eyes as they embrace proven acquisition and delivery systems that are reducing costs and improving access to their providers. We are seeing a clear and dramatic increase in the trend as more and more provider networks acknowledge and invest in the deployment of cost-cutting delivery systems across the US and around the world. The benefits of telemedicine are not lost on other countries, which are moving quickly to set up nationwide programs to serve their citizens.

Mobile Platforms and Affordability
In the immediate future, new products and services will allow health care providers to quickly obtain better patient medical imagery and data on the platform of their choice – a computer, tablet/iPad, Smartphone or other device. Innovative ways in which mobile platforms are being used to help revolutionize health care are already emerging. For example, GE Healthcare manufactures the Vscan, a portable ultrasound device that allows a physician to peer directly into a patient's heart, checking out the muscle, the valves, the rhythm and the blood flow. The patient can view everything at the same time. The Vscan, which is roughly the size of a cell phone, replaces the old-fashioned stethoscope and provides infinitely more information, leading to more informed decisions by doctors and patients.

GlobalMed, the Scottsdale, Arizona based company for which I am proud to be the director, is leading the way in developing innovative mobile solutions for health care providers. Our TransportAV™ LTR system is a wireless ambulance-monitoring and visualization system. It uses a small video camera, digital stethoscope and microphone mounted on a stretcher to transmit live images of the patient to the trauma team waiting in the hospital Emergency Room (ER). Paramedics and nurses in the ambulance can send close-up images of wounds, real-time video of the patient's response to various treatments and audio of heartbeats and respiration. This allows physicians and other medical personnel in the emergency room to see the patient for themselves, so they can begin formulating a treatment plan while the patient is en route, no matter how far away the ambulance is from the ER.

The TransportAV LTR system currently costs about $20,000 and a Vscan is $8,000, but as these and other devices are used by more and more clinicians, the per-unit cost will inevitably come down. This is a perfect example of free-market principles at work in the medical marketplace.

Serving the Underserved – Access to Specialty Care

Disparity in availability of quality health care is a real human issue. Because specialists tend to congregate in urban areas, many areas in our country are underserved. Access to specialty care is crucial for patients who suffer strokes or have cardiology problems, because those are the very patients who need timely attention. While about 20 percent of Americans live in rural communities, less than 10 percent of physicians practice in those communities (Rosenblatt & Hart, 2000). Rural residents must also drive longer distances to reach health care delivery sites. Telemedicine helps solve the time-distance problem, and also provides the right care for the right patient at the right time.

GlobalMed technologies, as well as the products of our industry partners within the ATA, are in demand around the world because health care disparity is a global problem. Significant advances are being made one system, one doctor and one patient at a time. Industry colleagues are in agreement that with the massive convergence of technologies in the delivery of health care, the next decade will be an amazing time for all involved; those providing health care and those receiving it.

About the Author

Joel E. Barthelemy's first high tech companies were in education, security software and semi-conductor processing. He formed GlobalMedia Group, LLC (DBA GlobalMed) in 2002, which designs, develops and delivers proven solutions worldwide to highly respected institutions. He attended both St. Cloud State as well as the University of Minnesota and received an honorable discharge as a non-commissioned officer from the United States Marine Corps in 1987.

Mr. Barthelemy served as a board member of the American Telemedicine Association (ATA), and was the 2011 Chair of the ATA Industry Council and now serves as on the Executive committee. He also served as a Director of the Visual Communications Industry Group, an industry think tank. He is the winner of the Ernst & Young Entrepreneur of the Year® 2011 award for the Desert Mountain Region for Technology.

References

Affordable Care Act. Office of Population Affairs. http://www.hhs.gov/opa/affordable-care-act/

Buy Vscan. GE Healthcare. http://vscanultrasound.gehealthcare.com/?utm_source=Google&utm_medium=ppc. Published 2011.

Few Americans Using 'E-' Medical Records. Harris Interactive. http://www.harrisinteractive.com/NewsRoom/HarrisPolls/tabid/447/mid/1508/articleId/414/ctl/ReadCustom%20Default/Default.aspx. Published 2010.

Globalmed Debuts Slimmer, Lighter Transport for Telemedical Ambulatory and Emergency Care. GlobalMed. http://www.globalmed.com/press-room/press-releases/2010/globalmed-debuts-slimmer-lighter-transportav-for-telemedical-ambulatory-and-emergency-care.php/ Published 2010.

Global Telehealth Market Set to Exceed $1 Billion by 2016. InMedica. http://in-medica.com/press-release/Global_Telehealth_Market_Set_to_Exceed_1_Billion_by_2016. Published 2011.

Pre-Existing Condition Insurance Plan. Health care.gov. http://www.health care.gov/law/features/choices/pre-existing-condition-insurance-plan/index.html. Published 2012.

Rosenblatt, R. & Hart, L. Physicians and Rural America. *Western Journal of Medicine.* 2000; 173(5): 348-351. Retrieved from http://www.ncbi.nlm.nih.gov/pmc/articles/PMC1071163/ (November 2000)

Telemedicine Defined. American Telemedicine Association. http://www.americantelemed.org/i4a/pages/index.cfm?pageid=3333. Accessed 2012.

Versel, N. VA Division Saves $742,000 with Telehealth. *InformationWeek.* http://www.informationweek.com/news/health care/mobile-wireless/232600447. Published 2012.

Secrets to Success for Telemedicine and Telehealth Programs

Ronald S. Weinstein, MD, FCAP, FATA, Ana Maria Lopez, MD, MPH, FACP, Anna R. Graham, MD, FCAP, and Gail R. Barker, PhD

What is Telemedicine?

Telemedicine is a special type of clinical service that leverages video imaging and information technologies, including telecommunications. It is the practice of medicine at a distance which has both expected and unexpected consequences. Many specialties of medicine can be practiced at a distance using such telemedicine technology, achieving excellent patient and provider satisfaction. Practicing medicine at a distance adds additional layers of complexity, but it also brings needed services to underserved populations and can save lives.

What is a Telehealth Program?

Telehealth is an umbrella term that covers telemedicine and non-MD services such as telenursing and telepharmacy. Often, people think of telemedicine services in terms of single services, such as telestroke or teleradiology. Several different categories of services, such as teleoncology and telenursing, may be aggregated into a telehealth program. In universities, telehealth programs may have an even larger footprint and can include translational research and distance education.

Historical Telemedicine Programs: Lessons Learned

Multi-specialty telemedicine practices as we know them today have been around since the1960s. Surges in telemedicine activity have seemingly come and gone.

The first multi-specialty telemedicine program was established in Boston in the mid- 1960's. John H. Knowles, MD, a legendary general director of the Massachusetts General Hospital (MGH), set up a microwave linkage between the MGH in Boston and Logan International Airport Medical Station for use by the first multi-specialty telemedicine program. The pioneering MGH-Logan Airport Medical Station telemedicine program was a part of an ambitious MGH community outreach program in the Boston area.

Kenneth Bird, MD, a fellow pulmonologist and colleague of Dr. Knowles', along with John Murphy, M.D., remotely operated the first multi-specialty telemedicine clinic, located at the Logan International Airport Medical Station. Dr. Bird served as the clinic's medical director and personally handled many of the telemedicine cases. Using the private MGH-Logan Airport Medical Station broadband telecommunications linkage, Dr. Bird could *see* walk-in patients in the MGH-Logan International Airport Medical Station clinic via video, while he was physically located 2.7 miles away. He could talk freely with a patient and carry out a remote physical examination with the aid of an on-site nurse, listening to heart sounds, breath sounds and bowel sounds using a specially-designed electronic stethoscope. Additionally, he could assess blood smears and urine sediments by *television microscopy*, the forerunner of telepathology. Thus, without leaving the MGH campus and thereby avoiding the late afternoon traffic converging on the Callahan Tunnel linking Boston to Logan International Airport and Boston's North Shore suburbs, Dr. Bird and his MGH colleagues oversaw the primary care and specialty care needs of over a thousand patients.

Because it received national recognition in the press and was actively promoted by the rapidly growing space industry, the pioneering

MGH-Logan International Airport telemedicine program had a role in the creation of several other early telemedicine programs. It was a successful model program at a highly prestigious institution. The fact that Harvard professors embraced telemedicine and were early adopters provided legitimacy for this innovative approach to health care delivery.

One such early program, patterned after the MGH-Logan International Airport Medical Station telemedicine program, was an ambitious NASA-Indian Health Service telemedicine program on an Indian Reservation in southern Arizona, near Tucson. NASA had adapted space medicine technologies for use in terrestrial environments and was interested in showcasing them. Their technology overlapped with the MGH technology. Another early program leveraging the MGH experience brought primary care services and emergency services to employees at a remote Phelps Dodge Company copper mine in southwest New Mexico. The telemedicine services for the copper mining personnel were provided by a group of primary care telephysicians located 80 miles away in Silver City, New Mexico. They were separated from the copper mine by a mountainous terrain. The NASA-Indian Health Service demonstration project was in operation for fewer than five years, abandoned by NASA, which cut off funding despite the impressive, well-documented successes of the program. Conversely, the New Mexico Phelps Dodge copper mine telemedicine program remained operational for over a quarter of a century, well into the late 1990s, using the same type of telemedicine equipment utilized by the MGH-Logan Airport Medical Station telemedicine program.

By the early 1970s, health care policy experts from around the world were flocking to the MGH to see the MGH-Logan International Airport

Medical Station telemedicine program and learn its secrets for success. The MGH became telemedicine's showcase. Other telemedicine programs popped up around the world. For some of them, the MGH program provided a virtual life-line.

What explains the MGH's invention of multi-specialty telemedicine? Why was linking the MGH to Logan International Airport by telemedicine a high priority? Personalities, professional ambitions, and overarching priorities all came into play.

The hospital director, John H. Knowles, M.D., played a very significant role in conceptualizing and then creating the MGH telemedicine program. Knowles was an extraordinarily charismatic physician and a natural leader who was widely admired. He had an expansive imagination and took on grand projects. His reputation preceded him wherever he went. Knowles helped transform the MGH from a 1950s-era staid inward-looking, elitist Ivy League bastion into a outward-looking, community-oriented center of excellence. He became hospital director at the young age of 35 and was the face of the MGH in the 1960s and early 1970s.

Why did an institution like the MGH go to the effort of creating and supporting a walk-in clinic at a nearby airport? Travel time was reduced for the clinics service providers. The telemedicine program was used for health maintenance programs for the Logan International Airport employees and to provide some emergency services. However, there were far greater challenges to meeting the health care needs of larger groups of patients in the Boston area at that time. Dr. Knowles was addressing these needs by creating large MGH neighborhood health centers, but without telemedicine.

The MGH-Logan International Airport Medical Station telemedicine program served two functions -- it brought medical services to the airport employees and travelers; and it highlighted the MGH's commitment to community outreach in a way that was highly visible and often newsworthy. This was appealing to Dr. Knowles since it cast his MGH community outreach programs in a very attractive light. Although the MGH-Logan International Airport Medical Station telemedicine program was one of several MGH community outreach programs at the time, it often topped the list of MGH community outreach programs in terms of national and international visibility.

The MGH-Logan International Airport Telemedicine Program also became a component of the MGH's institutional marketing strategy. The value added to the brand-name of a leading medical institution such as the MGH was enhanced by site-specific breakthroughs in technology and therapies. As an institution, MGH thrived on "made-here" innovations and lists of "firsts" in translational research and health care delivery. Both Dr. Knowles and his colleague Dr. Bird were exceptional marketers who personally thrived on being in the limelight.

With respect to MGH's telemedicine innovations, the emergence of copy-cat programs validated the pioneering aspects of MGH's work in telemedicine, with resultant ripple effects on other MGH clone-like programs. The 1970s decision of NASA to sponsor an ambitious telemedicine program in Arizona helped validate NASA's commitment to fostering the commercialization of technologies initially developed for their space program. It is noteworthy that the Phelps Dodge copper mine telemedicine program, modeled after the MGH-Logan International Airport Medical Station telemedicine program and duplicating many of the protocols used for the NASA-IHS-Indian

Reservation program, turned out to be the early multi-specialty telemedicine program that actually achieved long-term sustainability, remaining in service for over a quarter of a century. The Phelps Dodge telemedicine program has been largely overlooked by scholars in the telemedicine history field even though their telemedicine clinic in Southwest New Mexico was accessible to visitors.

Does initial success ensure long-term survivability of an academic program? It can be argued that the deck was somewhat stacked against the long term survivability of the MGH-Logan International Airport Medical Station telemedicine program. Dr. Knowles had higher ambitions beyond his general directorship of the MGH. When judged as a proof-of concept demonstration, the MGH-Logan Airport Medical Station telemedicine program was a success. However, the actual value of the immediate availability of health care services for maintenance of airport employee health care, in terms of patient outcomes, was apparently never put to the test. Some of the telemedicine patients were travelers who were lost to follow-up.

Oftentimes innovation trumps long-term stewardship in the hierarchy of academic values at high-quality learning institutions in the United States. All things being equal, top academic physicians are often better off starting their own programs from scratch rather than maintaining an existing program that is someone else's legacy. At the MGH, a clinical leader doesn't automatically get top billing for merely "maintaining" an existing program. Sometimes, highly innovative programs may be downsized or cease to exist when the principle innovators, or their administrative proponents move on.

The MGH-Logan Airport Medical Station telemedicine program may be a case in point. The program's champions faded away from the telemedicine scene by the mid-1970s. Dr. Knowles relocated to New York City to become President of the Rockefeller Foundation. He died at the height of his career, at age 52, from pancreatic cancer. Dr. Bird left telemedicine for personal reasons. By the year 1980, the MGH lifeline had disappeared. The world had gone nearly dark with respect to telemedicine, as the first wave of telemedicine programs had largely vanished. However, there were exceptions.

Why did the Phelps Dodge Company telemedicine program continue its operations for over 25 years, well into the late 1990s when it was lost to follow-up? First of all, it was of high value to the Phelps Dodge Company, filling a critical need for immediate access to health care services for workers in a hazardous industry. It was insulated from academia which can be an advantage for a corporation shunning publicity. Phelps Dodge telemedicine satisfied a mandate of the New Mexico Department of Health Services, which required an acceptable means of health services be provided to its copper mine personnel. Periodic audits by the New Mexico Department of Health Services validated the adequacy of telemedicine.

The Legacy of Health Care Innovations

There is often a fine line between promoting a new technology and overselling it. In order to understand the demise of the first wave of telemedicine activities, it is reasonable to ask whether telemedicine was oversold by Dr. Knowles and Dr. Bird. Or were these academic physicians, in fact, innovators who were simply ahead of their time?

We would suggest that Dr. Bird and Dr. Knowles left an indelible legacy that launched modern telemedicine and telehealth. Although there was a dramatic decline in telemedicine activities around the United States in the early 1980s, the MGH brand of telemedicine services remained active in people's thoughts and was discussed by health policy leaders for decades. Additionally, the first-wave of telemedicine programs inspired outstanding written scholarship by authors such as Rashid Bashshur, PhD, and Gary W. Shannon, PhD. Currently a distinguished professor-emeritus at the University of Michigan, Dr. Bashshur personally evaluated the original MGH-Logan International Airport Telemedicine Program on-site in the late 1960s. This was at the beginning of his career-long commitment to telemedicine, now spanning over 45 years. His scholarly writings serve as the "corporate memory" for the telemedicine field.

MGH Telemedicine "Knock-off" Programs

A second wave of telemedicine programs began in 1989 when the Texas state legislature funded a number of small telemedicine demonstration projects. Other states followed suit by developing statewide knock-off versions of the original MGH telemedicine program. Two second-generation programs were founded by former co-residents at the MGH during the Knowles-Bird era, Dr. Jay Sanders and Dr. Ronald S. Weinstein.

Georgia and Arizona were at the leading edge of the resurgence of telemedicine programs in the 1990's. The Georgia telemedicine program, founded in 1993 and directed by Dr. Sanders, became a multi-site telemedicine network that served as a model program which other multi-specialty programs then emulated. Although the Georgia program was significantly downsized in the late 1990s, it inspired interest and confidence among public policy leaders in other states in telemedicine technology, and created a desirable aura of success that gave leaders the sense that telemedicine had matured as a technology. Currently, Georgia once again has a large, rapidly growing state-wide telemedicine program.

The Arizona Telemedicine Program (ATP), co-founded in 1996 by Ronald S. Weinstein, MD and an influential Arizona State legislator, State Representative Robert "Bob" Burns, included critical components in their business plan to ensure sustainability of the ATP. In Arizona, commercial telecommunications companies were disinterested in the rural broadband telecommunications market in the 1990s. Thus, the ATP built out its own private telecommunications network. Sixteen years later, the Arizona Rural Telemedicine Network is still operated by the ATP's in-house corps of engineers and managed from within the University of Arizona in Tucson. It provides immediate availability of a level of information technology services unobtainable in the commercial telecommunications market in Arizona today.

The ATP also created an innovative membership-based Application Service Provider business model, which provides a level playing field for Arizona telemedicine for many health care organizations within the state. Fifty-five health care organizations, in both the public and private sectors, are members of the ATP, pay an annual membership fee, and use its telecommunications infrastructure. Telemedicine and telehealth services in over 60 medical specialties have been provided over the ATP's network by a number of independent service providers. There have been over one million telemedicine case encounters.

The ATP also has an innovative governance structure. This grew out of concerns over the priorities of a research university, which later proved to be well founded. In order to insure that the ATP remains a state-wide enterprise, and not an exclusive asset of the University of Arizona, a highly visible, blue ribbon Arizona Telemedicine Council (ATC) consisting of 25 public and private sector members was created. The ATC serves as a bridge between the ATP and the Arizona State Legislature. The ATC has met quarterly for 16 years on the campus of the Arizona State Legislature in Phoenix. Minutes from these two-hour meetings go to the Director of the Joint Legislative Budget Committee of the Arizona State House of Representatives and the Arizona State Senate for review. Arizona Representative Robert "Bob" Burns, co-founder of the Arizona Telemedicine Program, served many terms in the Arizona House of Representatives and eventually was elected to the State Senate, completing his legislative career as Senate President in 2009. Even after terming out of the state legislature, he has continued to serve as Chair of the ATC.

The ATP has shown steady growth as an academic program as well. It has participated in grants and contracts amounting to over $25 million in extramural funding. The ATP has been a fountainhead for innovations in clinical services, in translational research, and in distance education. This has been important to the sustainability of the ATP on a research university campus. The university expects its service units to be academically productive. Keeping the ATP at the leading edge of telemedicine and telehealth research, externally funded, and the recipient of a stream of academic kudos as a top program is viewed by the university leadership as being important to the long term sustainability of the ATP on the university campus.

Unfortunately, telemedicine and telehealth have yet to achieve *mainstream* status within most United States universities. Therefore, telemedicine program credibility can rest on the shoulders of senior faculty members with established track records of academic achievements in other areas.

Why Do Telehealth Programs Have a High Failure Rate?

One reason for failure of telemedicine and telehealth programs has been over-dependence on the program "champions." To avoid this pitfall, programs should have a leadership transition plan in place. The transition plan should be common knowledge to the leadership of the organization with buy-in. In addition, many health care professionals are unprepared for the complexities of ramping up a telehealth program. Jim Reid, a pioneer in the telemedicine field, once described telehealth as "four people running down a hall with their hair on fire." Practicing telemedicine is not easy. Professionals who have created and managed other demanding and sustainable clinical programs, and who are interested in taking on new challenges, may be particularly good candidates to take on telemedicine. Lack of experience in running complex health care programs can lead to failure. A telemedicine program is not the place to get entry-level experience in health care administration.

Another failure factor can be the misplacement of a telemedicine program within an organization. How many telemedicine programs have been assigned to the physician who simply "likes computers?" In general, we are skeptical of organization strategies that would place university telehealth programs administratively in non-clinical departments or colleges. Of course, there could be special circumstances, but as a general rule, this is not a good idea.

Basically, a telehealth service is a clinical service. Individuals managing clinical telehealth programs should be clinicians who possess the credentials to be clinical section chiefs or department chiefs. Their specialty is of lesser importance. However, it is important that the telehealth program's leaders understand concepts of standards-of-care as well as regulatory and reimbursement issues for medical practices.

The high failure rate of telehealth programs through the years is also related to the large number of telehealth programs that have been funded by start-up grants from extramural agencies. Programs initiated without sustainability plans are likely to fail. Literally hundreds of "demonstration projects" have been funded through various federal, state and not-for-profit agency programs. Such programs often collapse when the start-up funding ends.

A lesson learned is that telemedicine can be ill-suited to be a pilot project. Unsustainable telehealth projects can do more harm than good if they encourage reconfiguring traditional referral patterns and then abandon commitments without adequate notice of termination of their telehealth services.

What Increases the Odds for Success?

The likelihood of success is increased when telehealth provides:

1. **Gap service coverage**. Teleradiology is a heavily used service, driven by the needs of many small hospitals for night-time radiology service coverage. Large teaching institutions use teleradiology services provided by radiology department faculty members working from home for immediate "read-overs" of residents' night-time diagnoses.

2. **Urgent services**. There are a number of urgent services that are successfully covered by telemedicine.

Telestroke services are used during the "golden" one to three hours when administration of clot-busting drugs to patients can avert the progression into a stroke by alleviating the obstruction of a major brain blood vessel. Panels of teleneurologists may be on-call 24/7 to provide remote diagnostic services.

Teletrauma services have saved lives by providing doctors at small rural hospitals with telepresence advice for the management of patients. A trauma surgeon observes the activities on-going in an emergency room and provides advice on priority of services, while overseeing procedures, such as the passage of an endotracheal tube or the repair of a wounded neck blood vessel.

Teleburn services have been instituted in networks of hospitals, as burn care is a highly specialized field and expertise can be provided at a distance.

Electronic intensive care service units are becoming commonplace and have been instituted in a number of large health care systems. Teleintensive care nurses and telephysicians provide professional oversight of care from call centers.

3. **Mandated services**. Urgent psychiatric evaluations for non-voluntary institutionalization proceedings can be performed via telepsychiatry.

Additionally, the United States Supreme Court regards the denial of health services to prison inmates as "cruel and unusual punishment." As such, the Department of Corrections are required to provide mandated health services for inmates. Tens of thousands of inmates in many states, including Arizona, California, Iowa, Massachusetts, New York and Texas have received health care by telemedicine and telehealth for years.

What Decreases the Odds for Long-term Success?

There are a number of barriers to a successful telemedicine practice:

1. **Reimbursement**. Currently, reimbursement is problematic, although progress is being made with respect to both Medicare and Medicaid. Medicaid telemedicine reimbursement varies from state to state, though a dozen states have passed telemedicine parity legislation that requires insurance companies to reimburse physicians for telemedicine services at the same level of reimbursement as ordinary services.

2. **Credentialing**. This has been another moving target. Hospital accrediting agencies have flip-flopped on their credentialing requirements for doctors providing teleconsultations into hospitals.

3. **Interstate medical licensure**. Federal agencies, such as the US Department of Veterans Affairs, provide interstate medical licensure coverage for their physician employees for practice within their systems, which is effective in addressing this issue. Currently, non-governmental teleradiologists working for commercial teleradiology companies must often obtain multiple individual state medical licenses. However, several states, including California and New Mexico, offer physicians special telemedicine licenses, which reduce the hassle and cost of practicing from out-of-state.

4. **Telecommunications costs**. Rural broadband telecommunications linkages can be expensive. For example, a T1 line (broadband linkage) between a rural site and the nearest city can cost over $1,000 per month. The Universal Service Fund, administrated by the federal government, can offset some rural telecommunications costs, but the federal reimbursement process is cumbersome. Nevertheless, tens of millions of dollars in reimbursements have been received by rural hospitals.

5. **Equipment obsolescence.** Managing the costs of equipment upgrades can present a big challenge, especially for telemedicine programs initiated with non-renewable grants. The need for upgrades over time, as well as the inevitable emergence of new technologies, should be taken into account at the time a business model is being developed for a new telehealth or telemedicine program.

Other Challenges to Rural Telemedicine Programs

Telemedicine programs in rural areas can present challenges typically unanticipated by urban academic center health care system managers. These include:

1. **Rural professional mobility**. Many academics who want to promote the telemedicine enterprises that will benefit geographically underserved populations might not be aware of the ways professional mobility and staff turnover affect rural communities and their health care systems. For example, the turnover of C-suite managers can be disproportionately damaging for *critical access* rural hospitals. This can have an especially high impact on small hospitals that

are *one deep* at most in their C-suite ranks (i.e., CEO, CFO, CIO, etc.). Corporate memory can be short-lived in the face of high turnover rates. Of course, personnel turnover is variable from community to community. Some rural communities benefit from the career-long leadership of very talented individuals within the health care sector.

2. **Patient frustration.** Patient frustration can have a disproportionately high impact on pre-scheduled telemedicine clinics. Patients are less likely to complain about being in a crowded waiting room of a busy in-person clinic than they are waiting for the telephysician to appear on video monitor. The schedule for telemedicine clinics can be tight when the telephysician is providing services to sequential clinics, one after another, within a single block of time. However, telemedicine patients are often unaware of the fact that they are part of a decentralized patient group waiting in line for telehealth services. As frustrations mount, patients are less likely to show up for appointments. *No shows* are common in telemedicine practices.

3. **Destructive flexibility**. We all want to achieve a high level of patient satisfaction with the services we provide. On the other hand, total patient satisfaction and telehealth system efficiency can be at cross-purposes. For example, it is often unacceptable to let a patient's real-time teleconsultation appointment slip past a half hour for the sake of the patient's convenience. As a result, heavily booked teleclinics may experience unnecessary domino effects, with patient delays up and down the line, when even one telemedicine clinic appointment slips. A similar negative consequence can occur if

the telephysician is late for his or her teleclinic. The telemedicine service provider hub site and the multiple telemedicine spoke sites must try to keep their schedules in lockstep.

These are factors that can blindside conscientious planners of innovative health care delivery systems, who are accustomed to an urban culture and the luxury of having waiting rooms filled with expectant patients.

Overarching Concepts for Telehealth Clinics

Planning, multi-site coordination, and clinical efficiency are hallmarks of well-run telehealth operations. Functioning well in the "virtual world" requires a certain level of imagination in order to have all of the players visualize what is going on simultaneously at multiple geographically separated locations. The "if I don't see it, it doesn't exist" mentality can become a crisis for a decentralized program. Training is necessary in order to keep a telemedicine program operating at maximum efficiency. Both the staff and the patients of telehealth programs are well advised to appreciate the fact that telemedicine and telehealth can be far from business as usual.

About the Authors

Ronald S. Weinstein, MD, FCAP is the founding Director of the Arizona Telemedicine Program. He is a Massachusetts General Hospital-trained pathologist who worked at the MGH when the first multi-specialty telemedicine program was established. In 1968, he was in the first group of MGH residents to participate in telemedicine. While on a surgical pathology rotation with Harvard professor Robert E. Scully, M.D. at the MGH, he participated in some of the initial "television microscopy" cases originating from the MGH-Logan International Airport walk-in telemedicine clinic.

Television microscopy was the forerunner of "telepathology", a term coined by Dr. Weinstein decades later. Dr. Weinstein has had a career-long interest in issues related to quality assurance in medical service delivery programs. A leader in organized medicine, he has been president of six professional organizations including the American Telemedicine Association. Dr. Weinstein has received many honors and awards including the Lifetime Achievement Award of the Association for Pathology Informatics, and the Distinguished Service Award of the Arizona Medical Association (shared with Dr. Ana María López) for their work in telemedicine. Dr. Weinstein can be reached at ronaldw@u.arizona.edu or at 520-626-2971.

Ana María López MD, MPH, FACP, is the founding Medical Director of the Arizona Telemedicine Program. She is a medical oncologist, researcher and educator who has dedicated her work to the amelioration of health care disparities. She has a longstanding commitment to underserved populations and is dedicated to increasing access to high-quality medical specialty care to all communities. Her academic and clinical interests are focused on cancer prevention, specifically in the area of women's malignancies, and in the development of outreach programs. She is the Associate Dean for the Office of Outreach and Multicultural Affairs, and is a Professor of Medicine and Pathology for the College of Medicine at the University of Arizona. She is the Principal Investigator of several clinical and health service research studies. Dr. López is also the Governor of the Arizona Chapter of the American College of Physicians. Dr. López can be reached at alopez@azcc.arizona.edu or at 520-626-2271.

Dr. Anna R. Graham, M.D., FCAP, is Professor emeritus of Pathology at the University of Arizona College of Medicine and Scholar-in-Residence of the Arizona Telemedicine Program. Dr. Graham is a distinguished leader in organized medicine and is past-president of the American Society for Clinical Pathology. She has received the Lifetime Teaching Award of the Arizona College of Medicine. Dr. Graham is a thought leader in the fields of telemedicine and telepathology, and has personally signed out hundreds of *telepathology cases while on service. Dr. Graham can be reached at agraham@telemedicine.arizona.edu or at 520-626-7345.*

Gail R. Barker, PhD, works in the Finance Office for the Arizona Telemedicine Program and is a Senior Lecturer in the Mel and Enid Zuckerman College of Public Health. She is an expert on telemedicine reimbursement. She worked on developing the Arizona Telemedicine Program's business model and has helped obtain third party reimbursement for telemedicine services in Arizona. Dr. Barker has performed a number of cost-effectiveness studies in the area of telemedicine.

References

Bashshur, Rashid L, and Shannon, Gary W. *History of Telemedicine. Evolution, Contest and Transformation.* Mary Ann Liebert, Inc., 2009: pp. 239-314.

Merrell, Ronald C. *Telemedicine for Trauma, Emergencies, and Disaster Management*, Latifi, Rifat, Editor. Artech House, Boston; 2011: pp. 109-116.

User-Generated Images in Health Care

Neal Sikka, MD, Director of the Innovative Practice Section at the George Washington Medical Faculty Associates

The last decade has brought to the general public high-quality digital cameras, which have become increasingly affordable and accessible. Physicians have long used images taken of physical findings such as scars, wounds, rashes, and other diagnostic patient characteristics to train students, as well as to monitor the progression or recession of disease over time. In most cases, imaging has been controlled by the physician. Patients were not able to easily provide a high quality image that was useful as a diagnostic aid. However, over the last few years, that has changed significantly.

In 2007, Parks and Associates noted that 41 percent of US household owned a camera phone. The development of low-cost, high-quality digital cameras has given patients the tools to create images that may have medical utility. Today, patients can capture an image of an acute problem and transmit it to a provider. The provider can then make a visual diagnosis without having the patient come to a facility, potentially decreasing health care costs by reducing emergency department (ED) and outpatient visits.

Clinical and electronic health care paradigms are not yet in place to manage the opportunity that user-generated images may bring to health care. Similar to the development of other technologies for medicine, we must consider the many ramifications these images may have on our care delivery paradigm. For example, in1896, William Roentgen gave medicine the x-ray. The x-ray not only provided physicians with an non-surgical entry to view the body, but also changed views on personal privacy.

The x-ray was rapidly improved and lead to the development of powerful imaging modalities like Computer Tomography, Magnetic Resonance Imaging and Ultrasound. Each of these imaging modalities has revolutionized diagnostic testing for many diseases. They also each been found to have risks and benefits from a patient safety and diagnostic utility perspective. CT scans deliver significant radiation doses to patients, while MRI cannot be used if the patient has any kind of metal in their body. A CT scan may be a good test to evaluate for a subtle fracture, but the MRI is more useful to look for ligamentous injuries. The idea of integrating user-generated images into our system of patient care will have risks and benefits, and we will have to determine the most appropriate and effective use of these images.

We are entering an era where the patient is garnering more and more control of their health. This is readily seen in the exploding area of mobile health care. Giving patients mobility and connectivity through wireless devices is changing how patients think of their health, interact with the health care system and manage data. Similarly, physicians are adapting to rapidly changing technologies, and grappling with ways to integrate new tools into existing medical practices.

Soon there will be over 13,000 medical apps in the Apple App store. The majority of these are for medical reference, targeting medical students and clinicians. The second most common purpose of medical apps is general health and wellness. These apps allow patients to track their exercise activity, medications, or symptoms. In 2009, a Harris Interactive poll found that patients were very interested in using their mobile devices for diagnostics. Advances in mobile phone technology and their relative low cost have placed high quality cameras in the hands of vast numbers of consumers. Mobile phone market penetration is over 3.5 billion worldwide, with over 322 million US wireless subscribers, there is essentially 100 percent wireless penetration. Given this environment, it becomes important to examine the issue of user- generated images and their use in health care.

There are many potential applications for user-generated images in health care. For example, they can be used for store and forward telemedicine applications which are commonly used for teledermatology. These applications benefit a patient who might capture a camera phone image of their rash and send or bring the photo to the dermatologist for diagnosis. The store and forward concept can be used to evaluate a red eye, an acute wound, an abscess, or a chronic decubitus or extremity ulcer. This is often done when a wound care nurse works remotely with a supervising physician. A parallel application is the supervision of a resident physician who needs the input of a supervising physician in wound management or closure strategy. There are applications in the App store, like "Love My Skin" that allow users to upload cell phone images to track their moles.

Are user-generated images of high quality? There are many types of cell phones and variability in the quality of camera in those phones. We conducted a study to look at the quality of cell phone images we could collect in a cell phone camera based acute wound study in 2009. We found that the majority of cameras had a megapixel size of 3 MP or less. Still, in our study, we had an 85 percent agreement (kappa = 0.52) between our study physicians on image usability for a diagnosis (author's unpublished data). In another study on chronic lower extremity ulcers, the study physicians had a similar usability agreement of 82 percent

Cell phone cameras are rapidly improving. We can only imagine that image quality will improve as well. However, there may be mechanisms to provide control for and feedback to the user, guiding them to capture an optimal image. Some characteristics to consider are the lighting, the angle, the focal length, and motion artifact in the image. Fortunately, capturing additional digital images has a marginal cost, and many images of a problem can be sent. The future holds a great opportunity in plenoptic cameras that allow the receiver to focus an image on any point of the image using viewing software. Such advances in photography technology may take some of the variability out of images presented to physicians by their patients.

While there is great opportunity for improving patient care with user-generated images, there are also privacy and security concerns. Until a patient sends an image to a provider, there is no HIPAA concern. However, it is important for patients to understand that their phone may not be secure and that they are storing their own medical images on their device. Anyone who uses their phone may have access to those images. The HIPAA concerns arise in the secure storage of these images by clinicians. Will these images end up in the EMR? Can the EMR manage the potentially massive storage problem that could arise? Certified EMRs will have mechanisms to securely store image files. The clinician will need to determine which images are useful and require storage and which should be destroyed. It is important that they are destroyed properly, as images often have metadata tagged to them from the software in the patient's phone that may capture the exact location where the image was taken. The clinician should have a written policy and procedure regarding the handling of this process.

In addition to the privacy concerns with user-generated images, there is also a potential for malpractice liability. The use of patient images in telemedicine is so new, that we do not yet fully understand the risks associated user-generated images. However, the telemedicine literature using the analogous store and forward applications has shown that the practice can be low risk if used judiciously. These images are a great adjunct to providing patients with high quality, convenient care. Not only could this technology save someone from an unnecessary visit to the ER or office, it could also encourage appropriate visits at the first sign of a serious problem.

User-generated images are poised to make a large impact in the delivery of health care. Surely the demand for limited health care services will determine the best use for these images. Meaningful use criteria and HIPAA regulations may one day address the privacy and security concerns, but currently physicians are responsible for determining their own criteria for appropriate use of patient images. Risk mitigation will force the development of appropriate policy and procedures that safeguard patients and providers. The full potential of this technology in the medical sphere likewise remains to be seen.

About the Author

Dr. Sikka is a Board Certified Emergency Physician at The George Washington University Hospital and Director of the Innovative Practice Section at the GW Medical Faculty Associates. He oversees the GW MFA Telemedicine Communication Center, is the Emergency Department Information System Physician Application Manager and teaches a multi-disciplinary course at GW titled Innovations in Telemedicine: Mobile Health.

Dr. Sikka has been a faculty member of the Department of Emergency Medicine since 2003, a Fellow of the American College of Emergency Physicians, and a member of the American Telemedicine Association. He is currently working on applying telemedicine and mobile solutions to remote medical needs in the arena of acute emergency care. Specifically, he is researching how emergency triage can be better delivered through mobile technology. Other applications include telemedicine advice to ships at sea, to remote clinics and teams, as well as correctional facilities.

References

Braun, RP. Vecchietti, JL. Thomas, L. Prin, C. et. al. Telemedicine Wound Care Using a New Generation of Mobile Telephones. Arch Dermatol. 2005; 141:254-258. Tsai, H. Pong, Y. Liang, C. Lin, P. et. al.

Consumer Health Apps for Apple's iPhone. Mobile Health News. http://mobihealthnews.com/research/consumer-health-apps-for-apples-iphone.

National Study Reveals mHealth has Vast Appeal in America. Harris Interactive. http://www.harrisinteractive.com/NewsRoom/PressReleases/tabid/446/ctl/ReadCustom%20Default/mid/1506/ArticleId/107/Default.aspx. Published October 8, 2009.

Naked To The Bone: Medical Imaging in the Twentieth Century. Piscataway, NJ: Rutgers University Press MobiHealth News. 2011, September 22.

Teleconsultation by Using the Mobile Camera Phone for Remote Management of the Extremity Wound: A Pilot Study. *Ann Plast Surg.* 2004; 53(6): 584-587.

Wireless Quick Facts: Mid-Year Figures. CTIA – the Wireless Association. http://www.ctia.org/advocacy/research/index.cfm/aid/10323. Kevels, B. Published 1997.

The Doctor is Always In!

Jim Prendergast, CEO, HealthNow MD

Kent and Sue Scott had spent a nice Friday evening with their grandchildren. The only hiccup was that Kent had eaten an apple that evening and it was giving him a bout of heartburn that persisted throughout the night. At about 1am early Saturday morning, Kent awoke to unrelenting heartburn and decided it was time to take action. Did he call a doctor? Go to the urgent care center near his home or the emergency room? Nope, Kent grabbed a sleeping pill, another Tums and went back to bed. As he tossed and turned, Sue Scott remembered that they had purchased a membership to HealthNation that allowed them to call, e-mail or even video chat with a doctor 24 hours a day, 7 days a week. After much prodding, she convinced her husband to call HealthNation, and within eight minutes, a doctor had called back.

Kent stated several times he'd experienced this type of heartburn before and that he felt it would eventually pass. He even went so far as to promise that if he wasn't any better by morning, he would call his local doctor but had doubts that he would reach him since it was a Saturday. However, multiple issues uncovered over the course of the brief dialogue prompted Dr. Emran to advise Kent no less than three times to go directly to the ER as his symptoms were indicative of a possible heart attack. Eventually, Kent acquiesced and upon assessment in the emergency room, was admitted to the hospital with a diagnosis of cardiac event. A few hours later, Kent suffered a more severe heart attack and was told by the attending physician that had he not come in when he did, he would either have died or suffered severe heart damage.

According to Gallup, a 2010 study showed that 30 percent of the people polled stated that they had put off medical treatment due to the cost of accessing a doctor.This is up 50 percent since 2002. Twenty-one percent of those polled admitted to putting off a serious medical condition due to costs, a statistic that reflects an all-time high. A recent Commonwealth Fund study posted on the Health Affairs Web site, showed that 42 percent of self-described "sicker" American adults had cost-related access problems in the last year. The problems included not visiting a doctor, not filling a prescription, skipping doses of medication or not getting recommended care.

Kent Scott could have called a nurse hotline, called his doctor, gone to an urgent care or emergency room, but he didn't. Why? In his words, "I really wasn't worried and didn't think I needed to see a doctor. Even if I had, I have minimal health insurance so the ER was out of the question."

In today's world, people demand to talk to the source. We want fast, convenient and affordable answers to our everyday health care questions. In a day and age when nearly every question can be answered in seconds on the Internet, it is unfortunate that access to medical experts is more costly with longer wait times than ever. In some states it can take up to 30 days to see a primary care physician. For this reason and others, telephonic or video consultations between a doctor and patient are on the rise and proving to be very effective.

Telehealth or Telemedicine as some call it, has many applications that are essential for the future of health care. Rural clinics are able to communicate with regional hospitals. Doctors can collaborate with other doctors in real time. Patients are able to see specialists across the country from their local doctor's office and nurses at your local daycare center can video chat with a physician when your child is sick.

One of the fastest growing segments of telehealth is 24/7 patient-to-doctor access. Patients can access a doctor via telephone, e-mail or video where their interaction is recorded and stored in the patients

HIPPA compliant portal for easy access and review. Doctor visits can be inconvenient and costly. This deters many patients from seeking the care they need, even when they need it. Teleheath allows a patient to address their everyday health care needs, anytime, anywhere, for a fraction of the cost of a doctor visit, urgent care center or emergency room.

Telephonic or virtual visits to a doctor are most effectively used for cross-coverage consultations. If you have ever called to see your doctor and he/she is on vacation, out golfing or booked for several days (or even weeks) then you understand the need for cross-coverage consultations. Often this can be done with a physician assistant or partnering doctor unless they are booked or it's after hours.

The ability to speak to a doctor when a primary care physician is not available allows a patient to address their health care needs immediately, rather than put it off or go to an expensive alternative like the emergency room. In 2009, emergency department visits went up to 136 million from less than 124 million in 2008. That was an increase of nearly 10 percent. Many of these visits were the result of primary care physicians referring patients after hours. It is estimated that as high as 66 percent of all emergency room visits are non-emergencies with the vast majority of them for acute illnesses that can be diagnosed and prescribed over the phone. Furthermore, Telehealth physicians are trained to understand the limitations of a telephonic or video consultation and only diagnose and treat ailments that have proven to be effectively handled over the phone or video. Most of these "common" conditions represent 9 of the top 10 reasons patients seek medical treatment from our health care system:

- Allergies

- Bronchitis

- Pink Eye

- Sinusitis

- Earache

- Strep Throat

- Upper Respiratory Infection

- Sore Throat

- Urinary Tract Infection

Telehealth Advantages: Patients

Surveys conducted after thousands of consultations reveal a long list of potential benefits to the patient.

Working mothers often cite convenience as the top benefit. The ability to call a doctor any time without taking the kids out of school, finding child care or missing work is invaluable.

Cost and time savings also rank high among patients. Access fees can range from $0 to $50 per call with a median $35 fee. This is lower than the average copay and much less than the high cost of visiting a clinic or emergency room.

An often overlooked cost of a clinic visit is lost wages due to missing work or the lowered productivity due to a worker's absence.

"I am a nursing mother of a two-month-old infant. One day I woke up with the the chills, a fever and aching all over. I had intense pain when I would feed my daughter. I knew from other mothers that what I had was a breast infection. With my husband headed to work and a baby to take care of, it was all I could do to make a phone call much less go to the doctor. There was no way I would have made it out of the house that day. After a couple of hours I got the strength to dial the number I had saved in my cell phone to HealthNation. In 10 minutes a doctor called me back and asked about a dozen questions before he confirmed my infection diagnosis. He reassured me I could still nurse my baby throughout the sickness and prescribed antibiotics. He also recommened hot compesses and creams. My prescription was at my local Walgreens within 10 minutes."

- *Julie Kewin, Scottsdale Arizona, mother of 3.*

Additional patient benefits with telehealth include:

- Reduced chance of secondary infection from waiting room germs.

- Three times more time with a doctor on average than an in-person visit.

- Ability to get a second opinion with little hassle at a very low cost.

- Ability to discuss potential drug interactions without the hassle of going back to the doctors office.

- Access to health and nutritional advice from an MD without making an appointment.

- Faster access to treatment on nights and weekends to help reduce duration of illness.

According to HealthNow MD Patient surveys, patients using a telehealth service report that they are more comfortable asking additional health questions and more likely to seek a second opinion for themselves or a loved one. They note better flexibility by being able to be more proactive about their health care concerns, address illnesses quickly, and begin treatment within as little as an hour from the first sign of symptoms. Finally, many patients feel comforted by knowing they can talk to a doctor when the need arises. Telehealth gives patients choice and a level of control that has been sorely lacking in our health care system.

Telehealth Advantages: Doctors

"I joined a telehealth network because my full-time practice working the ER was becoming too hectic and less rewarding. I was no longer able to listen fully to patient complaints due to the rushed nature of seeing multiple patients at once. I was always being pressed to meet the criteria of insurance companies in order to be reimbursed and no longer able to practice the kind of medicine for which I had been trained."

-Dr. Muhammed Emran, Houston, TX.

Frustration with access times, insurance reimbursements and rising costs are not limited to patients. Most doctors who entered medicine did so to make a difference and improve lives. Our health care system has its challenges and good doctors are looking for more ways to reach more patients without sacrificing quality or valuable time with a patient. There are multiple ways a physician with these concerns can benefit from the emerging telehealth industry.

> **1. Join a network of physicians**. Like Dr. Emran, many physicians have joined telehealth networks to supplement their income and communicate with more patients while increasing the time they spend with families. Due to the ease and cost of access and the nature of ailments treated using telehealth, the majority of patients and doctors report a higher rate of satisfaction than with a traditional doctor visit.

> **2. Offer a Telehealth Service to patients**. Despite everyone's best wishes, no doctor can be available 24/7 to their patients. Although an answering service, nurse or physician assistant

can be very useful, it is much more convenient to speak with a doctor and be diagnosed and treated immediately, whenever possible. By providing a telehealth service to patients, doctors can offer cross-coverage consultations to handle minor health issues that do not require a costly visit. According to HealthNow MD survey results, these convenient consultations have been shown to improve patient satisfaction, loyalty and referrals. By allowing patients access to a doctor via telehealth, more time can be spent in clinic addressing patients with more serious health issues and chronic illnesses.

3. Join a network AND offer the service to patients. A growing trend we are seeing is not only the acceptance of telehealth, but doctors incorporating it into their practice. This allows a doctor to practice telehealth when available, therefore earning a consultation fee. This has resulted in patients contacting their physician more often since the cost and time demand is much lower. If the doctor passes on his patients call, the patient is then routed to another doctor in the network. This model is growing rapidly and poised to be a significant part of a family practice in the future.

In the beginning, telehealth was seen by many as a threat to the primary care physician. Nothing could be further from the truth. A telehealth network that is effectively administered and supported by suitable training is a primary care doctor's best friend. Patients are demanding faster and cheaper access when appropriate, and telehealth delivers just that.

Without the option to use telehealth, there is a chance that people will choose to do nothing or spend hours in a waiting room with a simple virus or sinus infection. These more traditional models of care can result in lower patient satisfaction, medical staff dissatisfaction, complaint management and ultimately a loss of clients and even employees. In the last five years, telephonic consultations have become more widely accepted as doctors come to realize it is highly effective at treating minor ailments and referring back to a patient's primary care provider when necessary. This reduces the day to day stress on a family practice, and gives patience the convenience and control they desire.

Telehealth: Future

According to the American Telemedicine Association, it is estimated that 73 million patients are covered in a managed care health insurance program. It is also estimated that health care reform, in its current state or similar, will add another 30-50 million Americans to our health care system. With access costs and access time continuing to increase, a decrease in medical school graduates and a system that is already overtaxed by too much need and too few providers, our health care system is in danger. When you also consider America's insatiable appetite for quick, easy access to information and services and a desire for choice and control, it is obvious to see that the demand for telehealth will continue to grow for years to come. According to Dr. Emran, Chief Medical Officer of Ameridoc and practicing telehealth physician, "The future for telemedicine is very bright because it reflects the willingness of doctors and patients to engage in meaningful conversations that are convenient to the patient and rewarding for the doctor. Health care laws are being revised to provide more holistic treatment plans to be developed with an effort on prevention of disease which includes access to medication refills for diabetes, hypertension, and high cholesterol. As younger physicians are being trained, they will gravitate towards technology and more open-minded approaches, providing higher quality care outside of the traditional 9 to 5 schedule."

As technology continues to improve and cell phones become more secure, mobile devices will allow video consultations, at-home monitoring and the transmission of vitals signs. This will allow telehealth providers to address more issues much faster and more cost efficiently than ever before. Doctors who choose to embrace this trend will reap the financial and lifestyle benefits telehealth affords.

Understanding the benefits of addressing a sinus infection from the comfort of your own home or being able to access a doctor in minutes, even when your thousands of mile from home on vacation is easy. But what about the nearly one in three people who put off medical treatment because of the high costs? What about the millions of people who simply suffer through their illness due to a lack of insurance or long wait times? What about the single mothers who do not have benefits and cannot provide even the basic care to their child with an ear infection? For those people, our system is costly, cumbersome, inconvenient and lacking resources. Telehealth can help them. Maybe even save their life.

About the Author

Jim is CEO of HealthNow MD a leading provider of telemedicine in the United States. Jim has spent 17 years creating, owning, and building companies. Additionally he has been a co-host of "The Block Where Wealth Happens," a radio show on the Financial News Network in Phoenix, Arizona. Jim has also been the keynote speaker for many local and national companies.

About The Thought Leaders Project

We live in a world full amazing people tackling incredible challenges. What happens when leaders go above and beyond to share this knowledge with their peers? How will you take these ideas and build upon them to become the next thought leader?

Progress and positive change.

We are helping to spread ideas of which we're proud.

Our core beliefs:

- Exceptionally high quality best practices and tips, created by those working in the trenches.
- Ideas packaged with urgency and action in mind. There is no room for filler.
- Powerful ideas and works spread. Create content that is invaluable when spread, and then package it so it's easy for others to benefit, grow and share.
- Reward those who stand up and spread these ideas and experiences.

Thank You...

For reading The Thought Leaders Project: E-Health, Telemedicine, Connected Health - The Next Wave of Medicine.

We would greatly appreciate your candid feedback about your experience with the book and would encourage you to express your opinions via a review on Amazon.com (http://bit.ly/TLP-Telemedicine), your blog, our other preferred channels of expression.

We welcome the good, the bad and the ugly.

Thank you again!

www.ingramcontent.com/pod-product-compliance
Lightning Source LLC
Chambersburg PA
CBHW051335170526
45166CB00002B/820